Integrated Delivery Systems

Ensuring Successful Physician–Hospital Partnerships

NICK A. FABRIZIO, PhD, FACMPE, FACHE

with Robert C. Bohlmann, FACMPE

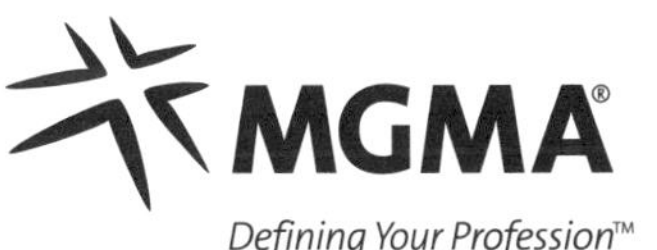

Production Credits
Publisher: Marilee Aust
Project Editor: Anne Serrano, MA
Developmental Editor: Bob Redling
Copy Editor: Katharine Dvorak
Composition: Virginia Howe
Proofreader: Mary Kay Kozyra
Indexer: Sara Lynn Eastler
Cover Design: Amy Kenreich

Library of Congress Cataloging-in-Publication Data
Fabrizio, Nick A.
Integrated delivery systems : ensuring successful physician-hospital partnerships / Nick A. Fabrizio, with Robert C. Bohlmann.
p. ; cm.
Includes bibliographical references and index.
Summary: "Describes how to build and operate a successful integrated delivery system. Whether you are running or bringing together hundreds of providers or merging two solo practitioner groups, this book guides you through the key issues of integration including structural, relational, planning, legal, operational, physician leadership, marketing, and technological considerations"--Provided by publisher.
ISBN 978-1-56829-342-4
1. Group medical practice. 2. Integrated delivery of health care. I. Bohlmann, Robert C. II. Medical Group Management Association. III. Title.
[DNLM: 1. Delivery of Health Care, Integrated--United States. W 84 AA1 F129i 2010]
R729.5.G6F33 2010
610.68--dc22

2009025200

Item: 9010
ISBN: 978-1-56829-342-4

Printed in the United States of America
10 9 8 7 6 5 4 3 2 1

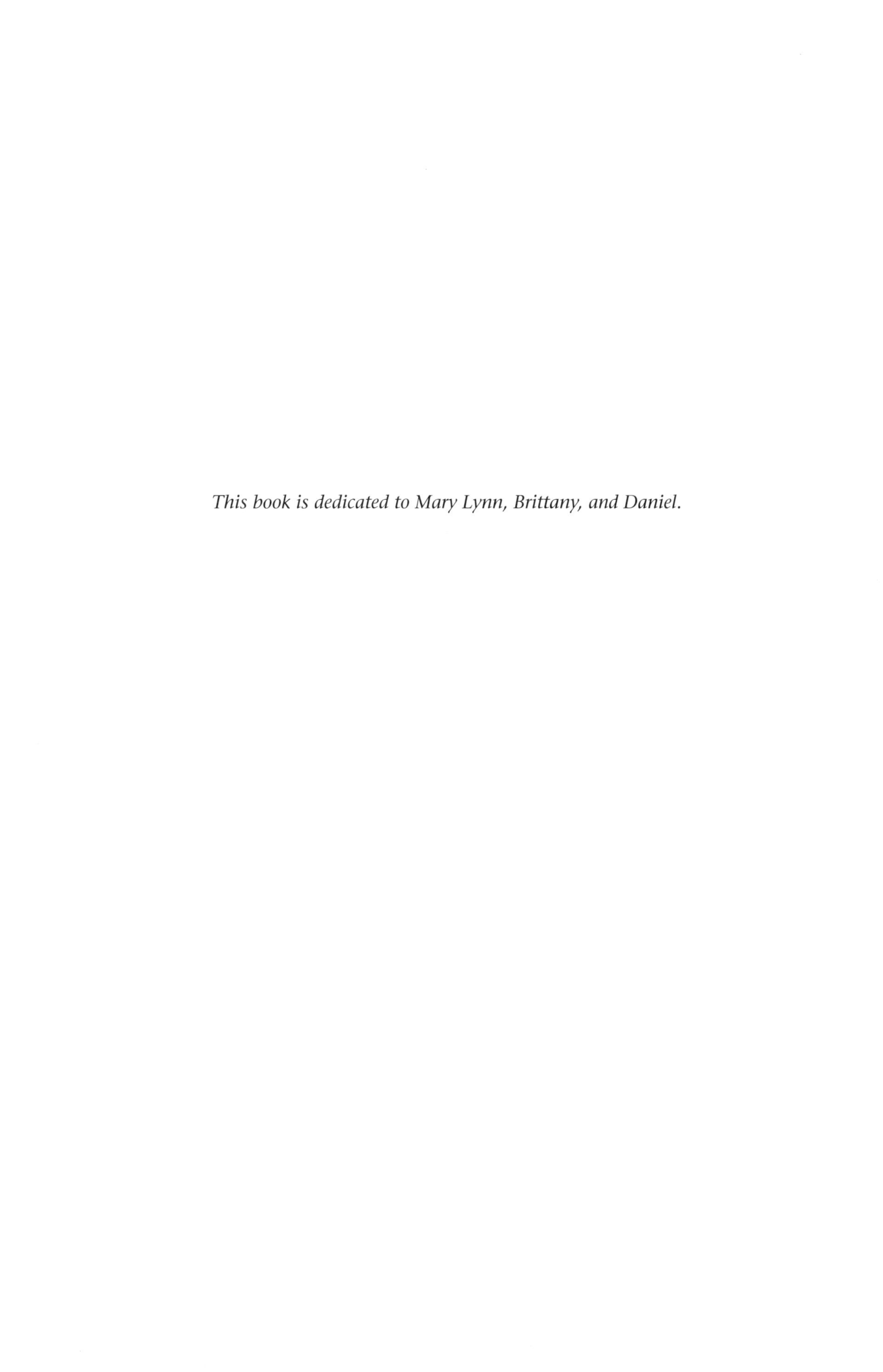

This book is dedicated to Mary Lynn, Brittany, and Daniel.

Contents

Preface

To survive and thrive in today's health care environment, health care providers must be increasingly competitive in this ever-changing environment. They face increasing pressures to maintain, build, or grow an infrastructure that can successfully navigate through and succeed the numerous governmental, regulatory, and service changes in health care. Health care providers also must deliver care in the most cost-effective manner while ensuring high quality.

In 2005, only 32 percent of physicians were in solo or two-physician practices, compared with 78 percent in 1975.[1] This trend is the by-product of providers merging with other providers and forming larger medical groups, and hospitals or health systems buying physician practices or forming a multitude of legal affiliations.

Integrated delivery systems (IDSs) are ultimately the outcome of such actions. IDSs come in many shapes and sizes, but their main purpose is to provide patients with the most accessible, highest quality of care delivered in an environment that is responsive and accessible to patients, and delivered in the most efficient and effective way.

In comparing the results from the 2003 and 2008 MGMA Cost Survey of group practices, we find that in 2003, there were 1,231 respondents to the Cost Survey and of those, 18.93 percent — fewer than one in five — were hospital-owned. In 2008, there were 1,470 respondents to the Cost Survey and 36.53 percent were hospital-owned.

This book will help you uncover ways to build and operate a successful IDS. Regardless of whether you are running or bringing together a group of hundreds of providers or merging two solo practitioner groups, this book will guide you through the key issues of integration including structural, relational, planning, legal, operational, physician leadership, marketing, and technological considerations. Several chapters are devoted to understanding the key components of physician issues, which is important for both physicians and executives. One chapter is written by a physician who has been involved with several successful integration efforts. Another chapter of this book discusses the pros and cons of the several IDS organizational structures.

The chapters are organized by key topic areas that relate to understanding both individual and group considerations that impact system success as well as the areas that must be considered when forming and operating an integrated system. The chapters are meant to guide you through the strategic, organizational, operational, and technical factors that are vital in both short-term and long-term success. This book also includes case studies, tools, and checklists that can help guide you in your own integration activities and due-diligence planning.

As medical groups, hospitals, and health systems position themselves for national health reform, they must be cautious in establishing relationships or affiliations because the concepts, implementation, and outcomes of integration efforts vary. From the thoughts and concepts discussed in this book, organizations should strive to articulate and work toward a common purpose and strive to communicate the concepts of integration in a pragmatic way that is meaningful to providers, administrators, and leaders in health care, and most of all, to patients.

REFERENCE

1. R. Cook, "Finances Driving Physicians Out of Solo Practice," *American Medical News* (Sept. 10, 2007).

Acknowledgments

I would like to thank all of the authors who contributed to this book. First and foremost, these are fine individuals who are dedicated to their families and communities. They are outstanding professionals whom I have either worked with or for. I have found each to be extremely dedicated to management, research, and improving the quality and delivery of health care.

Finally, a special thanks to Bob Redling who worked tirelessly with me on editing the chapters in this book. It was truly a national project!

CHAPTER ONE

How to Organize the Process

Nick A. Fabrizio, PhD, FACMPE, FACHE, and Robert C. Bohlmann, FACMPE

This book is written for leaders of health care systems that have either created, dissolved, or are considering forming an integrated health care delivery system. Our first challenge is to define an integrated delivery system (IDS). An IDS means different things to different people. It can be a combination of one or more medical practices that join together for many reasons, including increasing bargaining power, sharing resources, lowering overhead, achieving economies of scale, becoming more competitive, helping with recruitment and retention, or simply for survival. As you can see from this list, integration is a broad topic. In terms of the players, the IDS could be designed by hospital or health system executives or by an organization composed of mainly physicians that is led and controlled by physicians.

From looking at the for-profit and not-for-profit worlds, one thing is apparent in all successful mergers, acquisitions, or integration efforts: human considerations play the most important role in success. Behind the numerical, structural, legal, and financial considerations are people who must make the system work. The health care field is a much more difficult industry in which to merge or form organizations because groups must combine several independent practices and practice patterns to achieve true integration.

ECONOMIC TRENDS PUSHING INTEGRATION

Some of the economic trends that are prompting medical practices to merge or affiliate with larger entities include the consistent and unmanageable growth of health care expenditures. The Centers for Medicare & Medicaid Services (CMS) recently released projected health care expenditures for the 2005 through 2015 period. Total health expenditures in the United States are projected to rise to over $4 trillion in 2015. Per person health spending was $7,110 in 2006 and many project it will increase to top $12,000 by 2010.

Health spending continues to increase much faster than the overall economy, which is measured by the gross domestic product (GDP). Since 1970, health care spending has grown at an average annual rate of 9.9 percent, or about 2.5 percentage points faster than the GDP.[1]

Other factors contributing to the upswing in integration includes reimbursement stagnation or decline for hospitals, physicians, and other health care professionals. There are also new reimbursement models taking shape nationally including pay-for-performance (P4P) and cost management initiatives that encourage or discourage (depending on the stakeholder) the delivery of more efficient and effective care. The continued growth of the self-insured and uninsured is threatening the foundation of our country's prosperity, and Congress is sure to keep this on the agenda for the near term while pushing policies from Washington.

The expansion of services in the outpatient sector is forcing some hospitals to partner with physicians as more and more elective and ambulatory services are being performed out of the hospital. The growth in technological capabilities is also adding to the logical integration of services between hospitals and nursing homes and other large facilities with physicians. Technology is creating a more competitive landscape with the migration of more services being performed outside the United States. Notably, Blue Cross has allowed some policy-holders to travel abroad for their medical procedures.[2] It is possible that Blue Cross and other insurers would like to see more of their policyholders travel abroad for some of their medical care. As an example, a heart bypass that costs over $100,000 in the United States costs around $20,000 at some of the best private hospitals in Asia; $10,000 in India; and $18,500 in Singapore.[3] Some of these foreign hospitals are also accredited by the Joint Commission International, which is part of the same nonprofit organization that accredits many of the American institutions. As a response, we could choose to bury our head in the sand and say that our quality is better, but is it really? We could say that the care is better, but is it? We could say that we have better outcomes, but do we? Those tempted to say that exporting patients could never become widespread should speak to radiologists in the United States who are now in a very competitive landscape because competing radiologists from Asia, Australia, India, and Japan are performing several services for American institutions.

GOALS AND MOTIVATIONS OF INTEGRATION

As shown in Exhibit 1.1, various goals and motivations bring medical groups together. Some of the strategic motivations for integrating physician practices with each other and with hospitals include gaining advantage by having physicians and hospitals plan together strategically to capitalize on market opportunities and to reduce costs. Larger entities also have the advantages of access to larger amounts of capital, which can then be allocated for recruitment, retention, and other purposes. A larger health system also has advantages in differentiating the delivery system and providing increased visibility, which helps its marketing efforts and raises community awareness of its services. In other instances, aligning medical practices allows for the preservation of smaller practices in the community.

Along with the forms of competition from foreign-based health institutions comes another challenge — a crisis, in fact — that is related to the number of

EXHIBIT 1.1 ■ Typology: Goals and Motivations of Integration

HOSPITALS
- Create physician loyalties
- Market competitive
- Create external relationships
- Aggressive positioning
- Capture more health care dollars
- Short- and long-term survival
- Ability to retain providers
- Align mission and vision

PHYSICIANS
- Improve contracting ability
- Create efficiencies
- Provide more services to patients
- Capture more health care dollars
- Create relationships with other providers
- Provide pool of money for new equipment and technology

IDS

CONTROL OF MARKET
- Primary care base
- Specialty care services
- Comprehensive health care services
- Distribute services geographically
- Market effectively
- Bring new providers to community

NEW MARKET BEHAVIORS
- Shift of patients to ambulatory settings and outpatient services
- Hospitals and physicians creating joint venture opportunities
- Creating win-win opportunities
- Diversification of revenue sources
- Pooling of resources to make entities stronger

physicians entering the workforce. Today, a new generation of physicians is expressing that it values personal time as much as professional time. This new generation seems far less inclined to match the current generation of physicians' work pace of 80 hours per week at the office or in the hospital. Many smaller practices cannot compete in offering the benefits, manageable hours, and call coverage that their larger counterparts can.

Another consideration is that many more women are becoming physicians — up to 50 percent of today's graduating classes. Because female physicians raising young families are more likely than male physicians to seek part-time hours for a portion of their careers, today's smaller and independent medical practices face new challenges. In addition, many of today's graduating residents and fellows are not looking to become small business owners; they do not want to take call every other night and work 80 hours per week. And they have options to gain the work style they desire by becoming employees of a large health organization rather than shareholders in a small enterprise. This is not an indictment of today's newer physicians; it is merely a realization that health care is changing and those who lead it must change, too. These trends are a major contributing factor to the increased rate at which medical practices are combining and integrating with other practices and hospital and health systems.

Another motivating factor behind the movement to form integrated systems is to allow opportunities for hospital and physicians to create partnerships to expand service offerings, align incentives, share risk, and work toward common goals. Another aspect of combining strong medical groups is that while contributing to the advantages listed previously, the alliances also weaken the contracting, recruiting, and long-term sustainability of competitors.

Health care systems, individual hospitals, and physician groups have different motivations for why they want to form an IDS. The old saying "all health care is local" is certainly true for health care institutions.

Health care systems

Health care systems have various motivations and goals for developing an IDS, including increased power for negotiating and capturing market share. This can include a motivation to weaken the competition, which may or may not include other hospitals and physician practices. Certainly, physicians may be skeptical when one entity becomes too strong in a certain area. They may feel that it threatens their relationships and, potentially, infringes on the services they provide.

Health care systems also pose competitive threats to other health care systems and hospitals because capturing a critical mass of services and providers weakens the competitive positions of other non-aligned providers in the community and their ability to attract physicians, provide services, and use bargaining power with third-party payers. Many of these systems also have the advantage of a greater access to capital that allows them to link their member hospitals and medical groups with technology and electronic medical records (EMRs), which offer advantages that include increased efficiency, better connectivity, and the ability to measure quality and take part in P4P programs.

Many health care systems opt to offer services similar to those provided by management services organizations or provide a basket of options such as credentialing, billing and collection services, EMRs, and staffing support. Often one or more of these services appeal to local medical practices. These small offerings can serve as the catalyst for forming long-term relationships that, in turn, pave the way for establishing other relationships. Forming an IDS for the majority of health care systems is based mostly on gaining a competitive advantage rather than survival.

Hospitals

Hospitals share many of the same concerns as health care systems, but depending on the competition in the area, some interesting distinctions can be drawn based on the level and number of services hospitals provide and whether they are in a rural or urban area. Because health care is different in each community, many of today's rural hospitals struggle with physician recruitment and retention. As a result, the old-but-faithful employment model is re-gaining momentum in several rural communities across the country.

This trend — hospitals employing physicians — is also gaining ground in urban areas. It is still not as prevalent in larger metropolitan areas, but this is more indicative of the fact that many of those communities already have enough physicians so that there are other options a hospital can use besides employment to form health systems with physicians. Forming an IDS for many rural and medium-sized hospitals is based in large part on survival rather than gaining a competitive advantage. Medium to large-sized hospitals also have the advantage of greater access to capital and thus can link their inpatient and outpatient systems together to gain advantages in recruiting, measuring quality, P4P programs, and efficiency.

Single and multispecialty medical practices

Single and multispecialty medical practices often look at other factors that are important to preserve when deciding to form an IDS. While some of the same issues mentioned earlier about health care systems and hospitals are important, when physician practices look to merge with other physician practices, the most common issues to address include making certain that the right groups come together in terms of specialties, personalities, and quality. When physician practices join together, there is much more focus on making certain the same high quality of care can be provided by all physicians in that group. It's not that quality isn't important when hospitals and health systems look at integration strategies, but when physician groups look at mergers they usually focus on quality first and foremost.

Other advantages and disadvantages physician groups look at include the higher risk/reward ratio present in physician groups. Smaller medical groups have more limited access to capital, which often means that providers carry more of the risk personally if their investments should not pan out. This risk can be spread out by medium to large-sized hospitals and health care systems so that it is not the primary issue. On the flip side, if the merger and other service offerings are profitable, the reward is much greater for individual physician practices because physicians can retain most of those earnings without having to spread the wealth to other departments or services.

LIFE CYCLE AND STAGES

All organizations and service developments go through a developmental life cycle, and the same is true for an IDS. As shown in Exhibit 1.2, the IDS life cycle is filled with events that transition the organization from one stage to the next. Often, depending on how many groups have been integrated and for how long, the IDS may be in different stages at the same time.

In the *introduction* stage, the IDS is established and the alliances are formed. In this stage, the IDS is promoted through established channels in the health care community and the organizational values are linked with the business plan.

EXHIBIT 1.2 ■ IDS Life Cycle

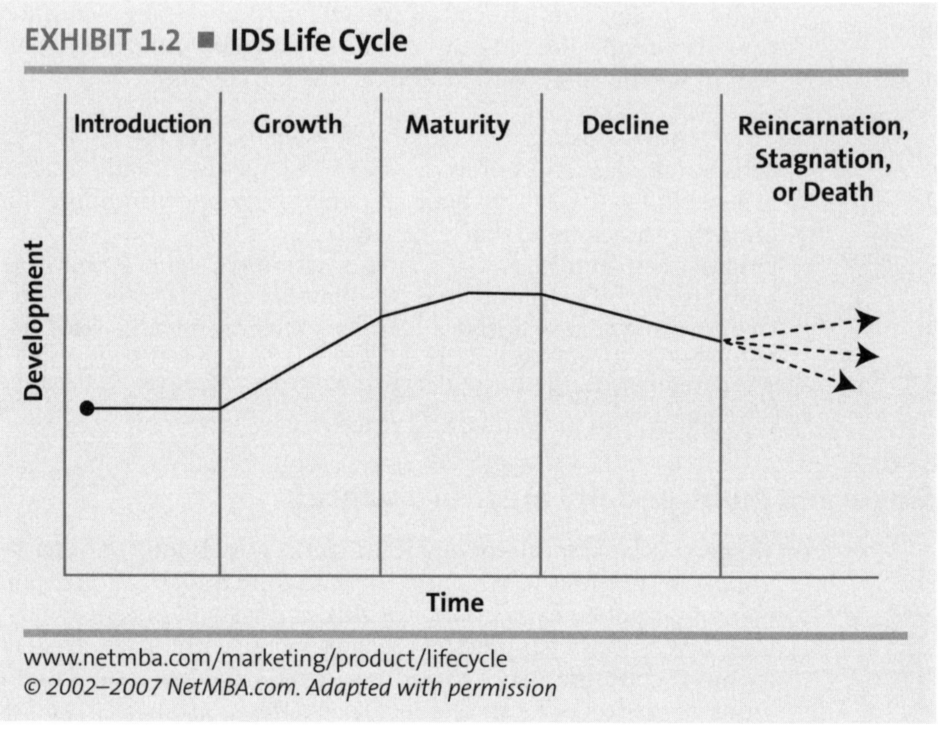

www.netmba.com/marketing/product/lifecycle
© 2002–2007 NetMBA.com. Adapted with permission

The IDS then moves through the *growth* stage during which the physicians focus on quality, making certain the IDS delivers high quality of care in order to advance its marketing and promotion efforts. In this stage, the IDS makes a strong push in its promotion efforts by trying to leverage its quality, service, and efficiencies through enhanced negotiations and favorable terms with insurance companies and vendors.

The IDS then moves into the *maturity* phase. In this phase it must differentiate itself from other providers within that community or be aware of competitors who may have learned about its success and may be trying to duplicate the model. At this stage, it is important for the IDS to maintain quality and emphasize competitive strengths and differentiate itself from the competition.

In one of the most important stages, the *decline* stage, the IDS must maintain its current strengths, improve on its weaknesses, address any gaps in service offerings, and discontinue any non-core or essential services. The goal in this stage is to reach the *reincarnation* stage during which the IDS continues to build on its strengths, improve relationships within the health care community, and address gaps in service and continues to improve the health care of the community while gaining market share.

The other options for this stage are much less desirable: stagnation or decline of the IDS. One of the hardest decisions leaders in the IDS may be forced to make in this stage is to discontinue or sell-off non-core assets or services in order to move capital into new service offerings. If the IDS operates primary care practices that are losing money, it will need to determine the worth of those

▪ CASE STUDY ▪

Transitioning a New Organization

Five years ago, Southlake Regional Internal Medicine P.C. (SRIM) merged two medium-sized internal medicine practices. It now has 25 internists and is approaching maturity. The practice recently decided to acquire a small (3 total physicians) cardiology practice that has been in existence for three years. The practice is relatively new to the area but delivers high-quality care. Clearly, SRIM is going to be very busy with transitioning this organization into the SRIM culture, but when combined it will also have an organization at the introductory stages of development. This is a challenge that the managing partner and the administrator will need to strategize over during the next several months.

practices relative to what they contribute to the total value chain through admissions, referrals, and ancillaries. The IDS must have an IT system that is able to track, measure, and monitor group performance. System leaders will either improve the system (*reincarnation*) and continue to build upon the strengths, maintain the status quo for a limited time (*stagnation*), or *decline*.

This is a point where most IDSs fail. The common belief is to continue to do what you started and have always done regardless of your current financial position, history, or future projections. To avoid stagnation or decline, the IDS must be nimble enough to move resources into new areas of development. Because an IDS consists of many parts, it is likely that some parts of the organization will move through these various stages at different times; the IDS must be able to manage the organization throughout different stages at the same time.

REFERENCES

1. C. Borger, et al., "Health Spending Projections Through 2015: Changes on the Horizon," Health Affairs Web Exclusive (February 22, 2006), www.healthaffairs.org (accessed March 9, 2009).
2. B. Einhorn, "Outsourcing the Patient," *BusinessWeek* (March 13, 2008), www.businessweek.com/magazine/content/08_12/b4076036777780.htm (accessed March 1, 2009).
3. J. Woodman. "Operation: Medical Tourism. An exerpt from 'Patients Beyond Borders,'" *Ability Magazine* (2007, issue 4). www.abilitymagazine.com/pbb.html (accessed March 9, 2009).

CHAPTER TWO

How to Structure the Organization

Nick A. Fabrizio, PhD, FACMPE, FACHE, and Bruce A. Johnson, JD, MPA

Many scholars and health care leaders who support integration efforts are of the view that the creation of an integrated delivery system (IDS) in which physicians, hospitals, and other key stakeholders are aligned within a single organizational structure, constitutes a fundamental strategy to address the current and impending challenges in health care. In early models, authors Coddington, Moore, and Fisher supported the notion that in order to effectively respond to changes in the health care marketplace, strengthening relationships between hospitals and physicians was paramount.[1] While integrating these two strong players in the health care delivery system was and still is challenging, many health care practitioners view this type of alignment as critical for long-term success.

The natural challenge in integrated systems is that the selected and/or elected leaders of the organization must manage relationships in both the hospital and physician worlds. These relationships may be based on sometimes competing perspectives and interests, and may involve powerful and influential stakeholders. Among others, these powerful stakeholders will typically ask a number of questions including:

- What are the key components of this integrated organization?
- What power, authority, and influence will each component enjoy?
- Who will control them?
- How much influence will they have on their respective pieces of the organization and how will that relate to the organization as a whole?

An integrated system and structure where roles, responsibilities, and authority are muddied, or where "leadership" within one or more components has little real authority, will be marginalized and lasting success will be limited. And because the establishment of an effective legal and organizational structure is essential to the integrated system's success, some of the other key questions that should be considered and discussed in connection with organizational design include the following:

- If the IDS is large and spread throughout several communities, how many distinct legal entities will comprise the entire integrated system, and what will be their respective roles, functions, and powers?
- Will formal governance be centralized or decentralized?
- Will the governance system be comprised, in part, of leaders in the community such as board members?
- What type of administrative and physician representation will be involved, and to what degree will the organization be physician led, managed, influenced, and controlled?
- What form of physician leadership will be involved, and will the organization have a strong physician leader?
- Will the physician leader have a management background or will the organization require that person to enroll in continuing management education?
- Will the management team of the IDS report to the health care system, hospital, both, or neither?
- What entity within the IDS will employ the management team?
- Will the IDS have a headquarters that is part of the hospital, part of a physician organization, within a broader health system, or somewhere else?

WHY STRUCTURE IS IMPORTANT

An important consideration when integrating physicians, hospitals, and other components of the health care delivery system is how to establish and provide legal and organizational structure to the organization. The old adage of form follows function is key in successful design and integration efforts. Organizations that are effectively integrated and aligned provide several strategic and operational advantages in the market such as greater efficiency and cost management, greater buying and negotiating power, and increased scale for information technology and quality-of-care solutions. Typically, in legal and organizational structures that are vertically integrated where physicians and hospitals coordinate services, several competitive advantages are realized because medical services are structured around a continuum of care — provided they are well managed.

While related and interdependent, an IDS's legal and organizational structures are not precisely the same. *Legal* structure refers to the particular forms of legal entities and relationships involved in the IDS and its participating providers of health care and related services. This includes the particular types, functions, and relationships between and among the separate legal entities that constitute the "integrated delivery system." It also includes consideration of the relationships — employment, service, and otherwise — between those components and the system's physicians, other care providers, and supporting staff. These issues related to legal structure will be influenced by many other legal considerations, such as those outlined in Chapter 3.

The IDS's legal structure provides the essential foundation for the integrated system. On this foundation is constructed the system's *organizational* structure, which provides the human framework and relationships within which the integrated system will thrive, stagnate, succeed, or fail. The organizational structure therefore includes the system's formal governance structure including boards, officers, and committees of the system and its component parts, as well as the management, supervision, and accountability structures within the organization. Whereas the legal structure focuses on forms of legal entities and the legal dimensions of relationships, the organizational structure goes beyond these dimensions to address governance, management, and other structures and relationships, and in doing so, focuses more on how the IDS actually acts and gets things done in furtherance of the organization's mission and goals.

BASIC LEGAL STRUCTURAL OPTIONS

Numerous legal structural models exist for integrating physicians and hospitals within a single delivery system. Each legal structural model is influenced by federal and state-specific legal requirements and opportunities, as well as by the organization's business and other goals. And while there are many different integrated system legal structures, several basic models predominate.

Management service organization

A management service organization (MSO) is an organization owned by a hospital, physician group, or other group of investors that provides management and/or administrative services to individual physicians or groups of practices. The MSO model is often considered one of the weakest forms of integration, but it is often used as a starting point for forming a relationship between hospitals, physician practices, and/or medical group(s). The MSO can also serve as the first step toward creating a more integrated, system as noted in many of the other structures and relationships described in the following sections.

In any legal structure, the hospital, health system parent, or other component of the integrated system can develop an affiliated MSO that can provide an array of services to physician practices. These structures can include physician practices that are already part of the system, such as the practices of physicians who are direct hospital employees, as well as those physician practices that are part of a subsidiary practice organization. But the MSO's services can also be provided to practices that are not formally part of the integrated system, including practices that remain wholly independent in the integrated system's market area.

The MSO can also contract with physician practices to provide them with services offered cafeteria-style, which may include one or more functions of the billing cycle, credentialing, and human resources including management, staffing, employing clinic staff, and providing salary and benefits. The MSO model typically involves at least a single legal entity — the entity created for the MSO itself — along with other legal entities that comprise the IDS.

▪ CASE STUDY ▪

Healthy Hospital and Healthy MSO

The chief executive officer (CEO) of Healthy Hospital spent the past few months meeting with several of the private practice groups in the area. Most of the physicians in the private practice groups commented on how difficult it was to run their practices and operate as small business owners. They liked their independence but did not like the business aspects of medicine. After several meetings with the physician leaders, the CEO of Healthy Hospital decided to provide the medical groups with services including billing and collections, staffing and human resources, and general accounting. The hospital created a separate corporation called Healthy MSO that was a subsidiary of the hospital but run by a separate management team including an executive director and billing manager. These two leaders managed a small staff that provided three key services to four medical practices in the community: staffing and human resources, billing and collections, and accounting. The medical groups paid a fee for each of the services they contracted with the MSO. After one year, the number of groups contracting with the MSO grew from four to six, and the consensus from the physicians was that they were pleased that the MSO provided cost-effective services that they could purchase to allow them more time for patient care.

Direct employment

Under direct employment models, physicians are direct employees of one or more hospitals within the IDS. The physician practice component is sometimes structured as an operating division within the hospital akin to other hospital departments, but from a legal perspective, the essential character of the physician–hospital relationship is that the physicians are direct employees of the hospital and not part of any separate legal organization. The physician practice operating division commonly has dedicated administrative leadership within the hospital management structure (for example, a vice president of physician services) and, increasingly, dedicated physician leadership.

As employees, the physicians have individual employment contracts with the hospital, each receives compensation in accordance with that employment agreement, each participates in hospital–employee benefits, and each is subject to legal and other restrictions relative to the hospital and his or her physician financial relationships and compensation practices. In the direct employment model, the IDS consists of one legal entity — the hospital — although additional legal entities can also be added and included within the organization.

Hospital-captive physician practice model

Some integrated systems include a hospital that directly owns and operates one or more physician practice organizations. Each such physician practice organization is housed as a separate legal entity that is owned or controlled by the hospital ("captive subsidiary"). The host hospital profits from the captive subsidiary and provides financial support payments to the subsidiary.

▪ CASE STUDY ▪

New Care Health System

Problem. Over the past few years, physician organization and hospital leaders in a medium-sized community noted that physician recruitment and retention was increasingly challenging. Many new physician recruits sought better quality of life and reduced financial risk and responsibility from what they could find in a traditional medical group practice. More senior physicians in the relatively large, 55-physician Community Medical Group were also seeking greater alignment with their traditional hospital partner. The physicians felt that a more integrated system would provide greater access to capital to invest in electronic health records and a better platform to respond to the demands of external payers. These physicians also had concerns about retaining physician practice autonomy and the unknown risks associated with becoming hospital employees.

Action. Through a series of informal discussions, physician leaders and the new senior administrative leadership of the hospital concluded that they shared common views. These included the view that the health care delivery system in the community was likely to require greater physician–hospital coordination and cooperation, along with new relationship models and ways of thinking. After preliminary discussions, these leaders decided to undertake a structured feasibility assessment. While many of the participants expressed a desire to move quickly to alternative relationship structures and models, the feasibility assessment was focused initially on helping providers more clearly define "what" the community needed (for example, business and other goals relative to health care). This step was deemed necessary before moving to the issue of "how" those goals might be structured and addressed in the form of new collaborative models and ways of working together. The outgrowth of the feasibility assessment was a conclusion that some form of a new system was both feasible and necessary, plus a fuller understanding of the shared and divergent goals, issues, and concerns that would impact the system's structure and operating format.

Planning. During the planning process a steering committee comprised of physician and hospital leaders and facilitated by expert advisors considered structure, governance, and relationship issues within the previously identified foundation of goals and issues. These structural issues were viewed as critical to address from the onset as they provided the framework for other key considerations related to operations and compensation. Addressing these structural issues also would provide a means to reach agreement on key issues before moving to more challenging questions relative to compensation.

Outcome. As a result of the planning process, the parties decided to develop and operate a new integrated system that would involve a legal structure comprised of a hospital, a physician organization, and a health system "parent" organization. This legal structure was viewed by all parties as critical to maintaining a sense of parity and balance between the hospital and physician organizations as co-equals within the delivery system, while also providing a health system parent to help coordinate the entire system via its strategic and ultimate decision-making authority. The structure was also designed to help promote local involvement and authority in the governance and operation of the physician organization — as opposed to being subservient to the hospital governance and management structure. The structure also would promote an enhanced sense of physician authority and sense of autonomy over the physician practice component within the new IDS.

Physicians are direct employees of the captive subsidiary, and the entity may function as a true "group practice" or, more commonly, as collective clinics through which physician employees work. Each captive subsidiary may have its own local administrative leadership. The system may have a single vice president for physician services who may or may not be a physician.

The form of these captive subsidiary legal entities varies based upon state laws and the IDS's business objectives, but the type of legal entities that are considered are typically limited to single-member limited liability companies (LLCs) in which the hospital is the sole LLC member, non-profit corporations, or even for-profit corporations (to potentially include various forms of professional practice entities where permitted by state law) that function as a physician practice entity. The hospital-captive physician practice model consists of a minimum of two separate legal entities: the hospital and the captive subsidiary.

Health system parent-subsidiary model

Under the health system parent-subsidiary model, a health system functions as the sole owner or member of one or more hospitals and a subsidiary physician practice legal entity, such that the physician practice is a subsidiary of the health system parent ("health system subsidiary"), rather than a subsidiary of the hospital itself. The hospital and physician practice legal entities within the IDS constitute brother/sister organizations subject to the coordination and ultimate control of the health system parent. The entire combination of legal entities — parent, brother, and sister —constitutes the IDS.

Given that multiple legal entities are involved, the health system parent-subsidiary model often has its own dedicated governance, leadership, and management structures. Financial support payments are frequently paid from the health system to the subsidiary practice entity, and the health system subsidiary is able to function as a true group practice or operate separate clinics that are staffed by the subsidiary's physician employees. In its most basic form, this IDS legal structure involves three separate legal entities: parent, hospital, and practice organization.

WHAT LEGAL AND ORGANIZATIONAL STRUCTURE IS RIGHT FOR US?

It depends! There are numerous legal and other considerations that must be considered before forming an IDS. Certain legal issues and options depend on the state where the practices, hospital, or system are located. Other equally important considerations are based on the economics of the community and the finances, experiences, and motivations of the parties seeking to form the system.

Many physicians who are considering forming or joining an existing IDS are influenced by what their colleagues in other communities or states have done, and their decisions will likely be based on the perceived good or bad experiences those colleagues have faced. For better or for worse, these stories — good, bad, or indifferent — often influence the way physicians think their experience with integration will turn out. For example, if a group of cardiologists in Alabama is considering affiliating with a hospital in their community, they may draw on the outcomes — good or bad — from their colleagues in other states. The danger in doing this is that while physicians in the same specialty provide the same services as each other, their outcomes could be completely different. This is due to several factors including their practice's current organizational structure, culture, overhead, staffing utilization, provider productivity, payer contracts, and several other organizational factors — including the people involved. The danger with using other groups' experiences as the "cookie cutter" approach to any new relationship is that it can either kill or hasten integration efforts. All health care communities are different, and several internal and external factors must be considered when forming an IDS.

GOALS AND NEEDS AS KEY DRIVERS OF STRUCTURE AND STRATEGY

Experience suggests that an integrated system's legal and organizational form should optimally follow the system's mission, function, goals, and business needs. Common objectives that drive the legal and organizational structures used in integrated systems include:

- Ensuring that the mission, vision, and goals of the integration efforts are acceptable to each partner;
- Ensuring that physicians can, and do, have an active role in the physician practice component of the delivery system;
- Promoting physician leadership, sense of identity, and autonomy within the IDS;
- Enhancing physician practice operations and management focus, and information transparency;
- Facilitating effective physician practice operations, including physician organization–specific human resources administration functions, compensation, revenue cycle management, and other practices;
- Providing flexibility to access hospital-based and freestanding physician practice reimbursement rules and compensation practices; and
- Creating flexibility in employee benefit structures.

How these and other business goals and objectives are translated into structure is frequently influenced by perceptions regarding the existing structure's strengths, weaknesses, operating experiences, and culture.

By illustration, while direct employment by hospitals may be a model that is available and administratively convenient in many communities, many integrated systems elect to create an entirely new legal and organizational structure for the physician practice component. The use of an entirely new legal entity is sometimes required as a matter of law (for example, due to state laws prohibiting physicians from becoming direct employees of a hospital or other nonphysician-owned practice entities). However, in most communities there are many legal means to the end — any number of legal structural alternatives may be used for a new or established IDS.

Despite the availability of several options, many systems make a business decision to use a separate-yet-aligned legal entity for the IDS's physician practice activities. The reasons for making this legal structural decision are numerous, including promoting greater physician practice operational autonomy. Sometimes, a separate-yet-aligned legal entity is created to help physician practices break free from a hospital environment's cultural limitations and administrative practices. Thus, the IDS might create a truly new legal entity and organizational structure in law and in fact, and with those, new management structures, financial management, and other operating systems. Creating something new is viewed as a means to help enhance future success.

LEGAL STRUCTURE, GOVERNANCE, AND LEADERSHIP SYSTEMS

Each of the three primary legal structural options for integrated systems — direct employment, captive subsidiary, and health system subsidiary — has implications for the existing and available governance and leadership structures and relationships. For example, under the direct employment model, the hospital board and existing management structure will typically continue to function as the leadership of the entire IDS. The IDS will commonly name a vice president of physician services or use a similar title for a position with a physician practice perspective that would organize and redeploy hospital resources and infrastructure in support of the IDS's physician practices.

Conversely, in the health system subsidiary model, duplicate board and administrative structures are commonly required. The separate physician organization subsidiary legal entity will have a separate board of directors — although there may be some, or even total, overlap of board membership with the health system parent and/or hospital boards. Likewise, a dedicated management structure is typically required to focus attention on the physician practice entity, along with health system subsidiary practice entity–specific strategic and financial plans, budgets, and other systems.

The governance and management structures used in the captive subsidiary model will commonly constitute a blend of the other two models. The captive subsidiary will commonly have its own board and management team, although those teams will more frequently track directly with members of the hospital's existing leadership structure.

PHYSICIAN INFLUENCE IN ALTERNATIVE LEGAL STRUCTURES

The legal structural options also vary in terms of how physicians provide input and influence within the organization. Under the direct employment model, physician influence will commonly be exercised informally through "operations committees" or similar bodies that provide input on clinical practice, operations, and other matters. Similar operations committees may also be used in the captive subsidiary model, although the committees will commonly focus on the operations of one or more individual physician practices in order to promote physician involvement in budgets, staffing, scheduling, and other practice-specific issues. Advisory boards and similar bodies may also be used to provide input to the captive subsidiary's administrative leadership or board regarding strategy, quality, and other issues.

The health system subsidiary legal structure may provide the greatest flexibility in terms of the range of potential opportunities for physician involvement and participation. In these systems, physicians may (but need not be required to) have a more active role in the enterprise's formal governance structure — subject at all times to the health system parent's "reserve" powers. In these structures physicians commonly hold a seat at the governance table, though the defined powers of the board will also vary from one system to another. Common structures will usually blend operations-specific committees that focus on individual physician practice operations with one more physician advisory councils to provide input to the health system subsidiary's management and board regarding physician organization–specific strategy such as quality.

THINKING ABOUT ORGANIZATIONAL STRUCTURE

Once the IDS has secured its legal structure, existing organizational and management reporting structures may need to be addressed and revised. Considering and reviewing the system's organizational structure — the governance, management, reporting, and other activities and relationships involved in the IDS — is also a continuous task, and each leader should routinely evaluate ways to make the organization more responsive. Looking at the way the system acts and reacts and how people within that system interact is a key management responsibility.

Depending on how long an IDS has been in place, or where it is on the IDS life cycle, some organizations will perform better than others. The physician practices, hospitals, and health care systems that come together in an IDS must also determine how much management (administration) they need to operate the newly formed system. Clearly, experience in managing medical groups is key in running medical practices. When hospitals bought and ran physician practices starting in the early 1990s, they soon learned that using their hospital managers or service line administrators to manage the physician practices produced poor results. Running today's medical practice requires dedication, support, and experience in medical group practice management.

SIZE, SCOPE, AND SKILL LEVEL

If two or more medical groups join together and the medical groups are small to medium-sized groups (15 to 20 total physicians), there should not be a need to have more than one administrator for the physician component of the newly formed IDS. This is the point where some economies of scale can be realized provided there are enough personnel to manage the strategic, operational, and financial responsibilities of the organization. The organization will also need to consider how many employees each manager can reasonably and effectively manage. Depending on the overall size of the organization, including how many sites are being managed and the total number of employees, the organization may need to separate out its clinical from non-clinical staff and have them report to different managers.

Many organizations err in thinking that managers with mostly clinical skills (nurse managers) can effectively manage the entire office, including the non-clinical staff, and general administrative duties without also having considerable experience in managing non-clinical staff and the business operations of the medical group. On the other hand, many organizations carry that same faulty logic to the opposite extreme and believe that non-clinical managers or those with management degrees can effectively manage nurses and ancillary staff. This is where one will have to take an inventory of the size and scope of the organization and break people out into clinical and non-clinical staff structures. The next step is to determine how many managers are needed and whether they must have the skills to manage both the clinical and non-clinical staff, the number of employees they must manage, and whether they have the competencies to manage the job functions assigned to them.

Other important considerations will have an impact on how many layers of management are designated and how the organization will be structured. These several factors include the IDS mission, the future environment, the state of the internal operations of the entities, and the culture of the IDS. The IDS will need to determine the level of importance to place on teamwork and whether the IDS structure will change the way people work. These changes could include creating cross-functional reporting relationships and cross-training of staff members. Attention must also be paid to whether the system will place a value on staff members working collaboratively to achieve results. (Later chapters in this book are devoted to the importance of the internal operations, culture, and organizational dynamics of the IDS.)

FORM FOLLOWS FUNCTION IN ORGANIZATIONAL STRUCTURE

An IDS must consider its goals, reporting relationships, and overall organizational design framework. This framework will determine how the system acts and reacts to change. As such, the design must be adjusted to fit the individual needs of the organization.

One of the first considerations that must be made is the organization's management framework. Some refer to this framework as the *span of control, span of management,* or *span of authority*. The central questions to be answered are: what relationship the supervisor has on subordinates, how many supervisors each subordinate has, and how many subordinates each supervisor manages. There are widely differing opinions among management experts as to the exact number of employees each manager can effectively supervise. This number is also based on how many supervisors each employee has — for instance, in a matrix organization, an employee may have multiple bosses. This is also the case in many academic departments where clinical faculty may have a divisional leader, such as the director of research or medical director for their ambulatory clinic, and the chair of a department who is also their supervisor. An academic department chair may report to both a service line administrator in the hospital and to the dean of the medical school.

Many scholars believe that the number of employees each supervisor can effectively manage can range from 8 to 15. Other factors that influence this decision include the following:

- Whether the employees are clinical or non-clinical (type of work);
- Where the employees are located (geographical location);

- The supervisor's qualifications;
- The availability of staff (competitive environment);
- The stability of the organization (turnover rates);
- The culture, climate, and values of the organization (Is it a nice place to work and do employees feel valued, respected, and compensated appropriately?);
- The volume of work (employees and managers); and
- Whether the organization is new (start up) or established.

Organizations often transform their organizational design or structure based on whether they have merged with another entity, acquired one or more entities, or divested and become smaller. Several reasons for this transformation to occur include more staff to manage, increased size and scale of operations, or the downsizing of offices, providers, and staff. Organizations must be nimble enough to adapt to the forces of change.

A conceptual view of the organizational design framework is shown in Exhibit 2.1. This figure illustrates the internal and external factors that influence organizational change. Leaders must have the skills and competencies to manage these factors and guide the organization through this fluid change process. Practitioners often want to move to the bottom of the framework and begin process improvement strategies, but real transformation and the success of strategic management lie at the top with aligning the mission and vision with the organization's environment, resources, and actions.

TRADITIONAL ORGANIZATIONAL CHART

The majority of medium-sized medical group practices (15 to 20 total physicians) have a variation of the organizational chart shown in Exhibit 2.2. Smaller organizations may not have the nurse manager position as indicated in this chart and larger organizations may have an additional director of finance or operations who reports to the administrator. These choices are mostly factors of size and scope. In this traditional organizational structure, the office staff (non-clinical) reports to the administrator and the nurses report to the nurse manager.

DEPARTMENTAL VIEW

The classical view of defining work is that work should be executed on the one hand and integrated and coordinated on the other. Management theorists subscribe to the notion that a relationship exists between integrating and coordinating work and completing tasks with the goal of achieving satisfactory outcomes. The concept of departmentation was borne by these early theorists, and this notion satisfies, in part, both of these requirements. Many of today's business and medical practice leaders have taken this initial concept and organized work into departments where tasks are grouped by expertise or function while individuals are assigned to those tasks according to their familiarity with that department or the activities of that department. The notion of

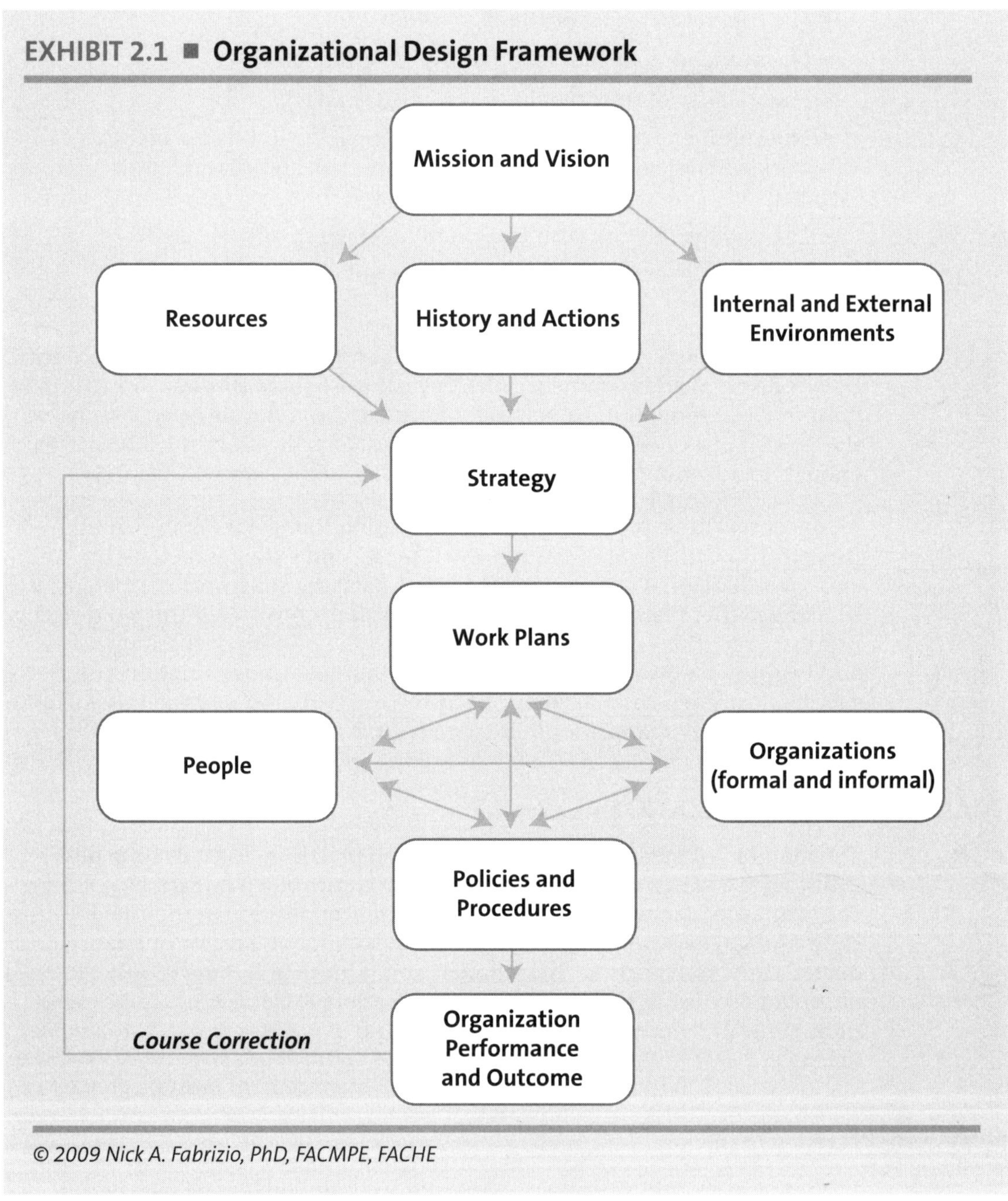

departmentalization is based on work being specialized by expertise and then an appropriate organizational structure, either tall or flat, is built around those work processes.

Several of today's offshoots to organizational design and structure are based on departmentation and modifications of the *tall* and *flat* organizational structures. Exhibits 2.3 and 2.4 illustrate the level of hierarchy in tall and flat organizational structures, respectively.

EXHIBIT 2.2 ■ Traditional Organizational Chart for a Medium-sized Medical Group

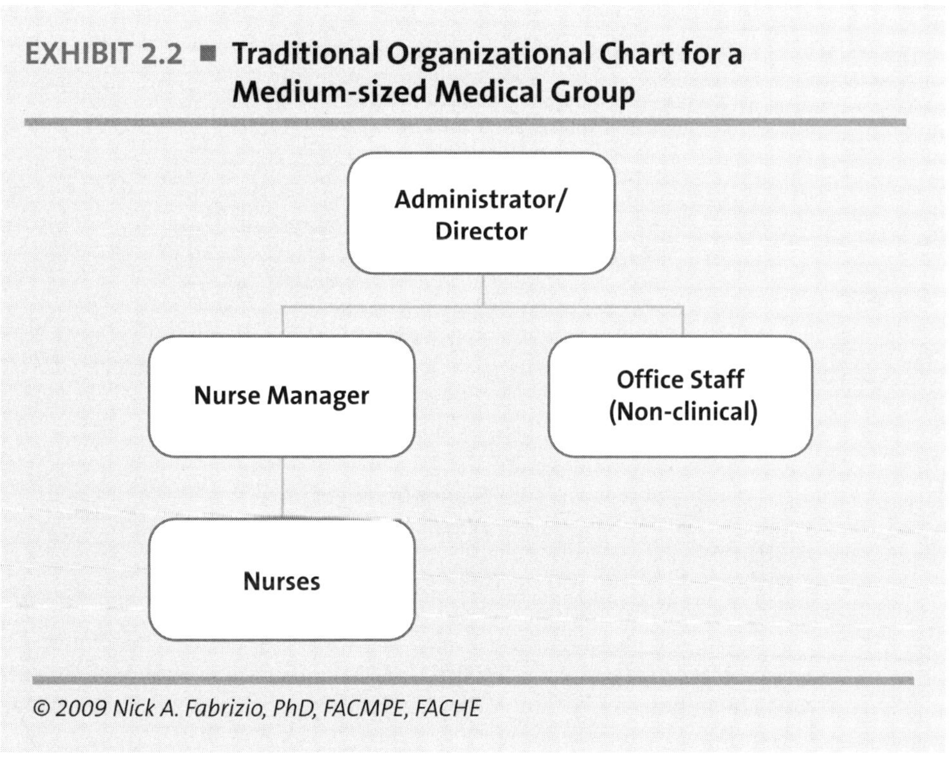

© 2009 Nick A. Fabrizio, PhD, FACMPE, FACHE

A tall organizational structure (Exhibit 2.3) may be better suited for a large IDS with several departments. There is more bureaucracy associated with a taller organizational structure, however, because tall structures tend to have multiple levels of supervisors according to the size and complexity of the department. In addition, as the number of supervisors increases, the potential for competing interests and projects increase and slow the speed of decision making, which is the antithesis to the mode of operation in private practice medical groups today. In tall structures there are more layers of management between the front-line workers and the senior managers, so often there is a disconnect between what is happening within the medical practice and the decisions being made. Clearly, this is not the case for all organizations with a tall structure, but as Exhibit 2.3 illustrates, several layers of management must be crossed to get from the lower to the higher levels.

A flat organizational structure (Exhibit 2.4), which may be present in small to medium-sized organizations or large organizations that have smaller departments, has several advantages. These advantages can be attributed to fewer levels of authority or bureaucracy and a more efficient structure in terms of noticing, reporting, and correcting problems. There are fewer layers of management between the front-line office workers and the senior managers, so these managers often have a better understanding of what "happens on the shop floor" and can more effectively communicate with the CEO. Some CEOs favor the flat approach as it allows them to be more in touch with the clinical enterprise. The flat structure mandates that the practice/service line managers are highly skilled and can function in a high capacity in both working with the

EXHIBIT 2.3 ■ Tall Organizational Structure*

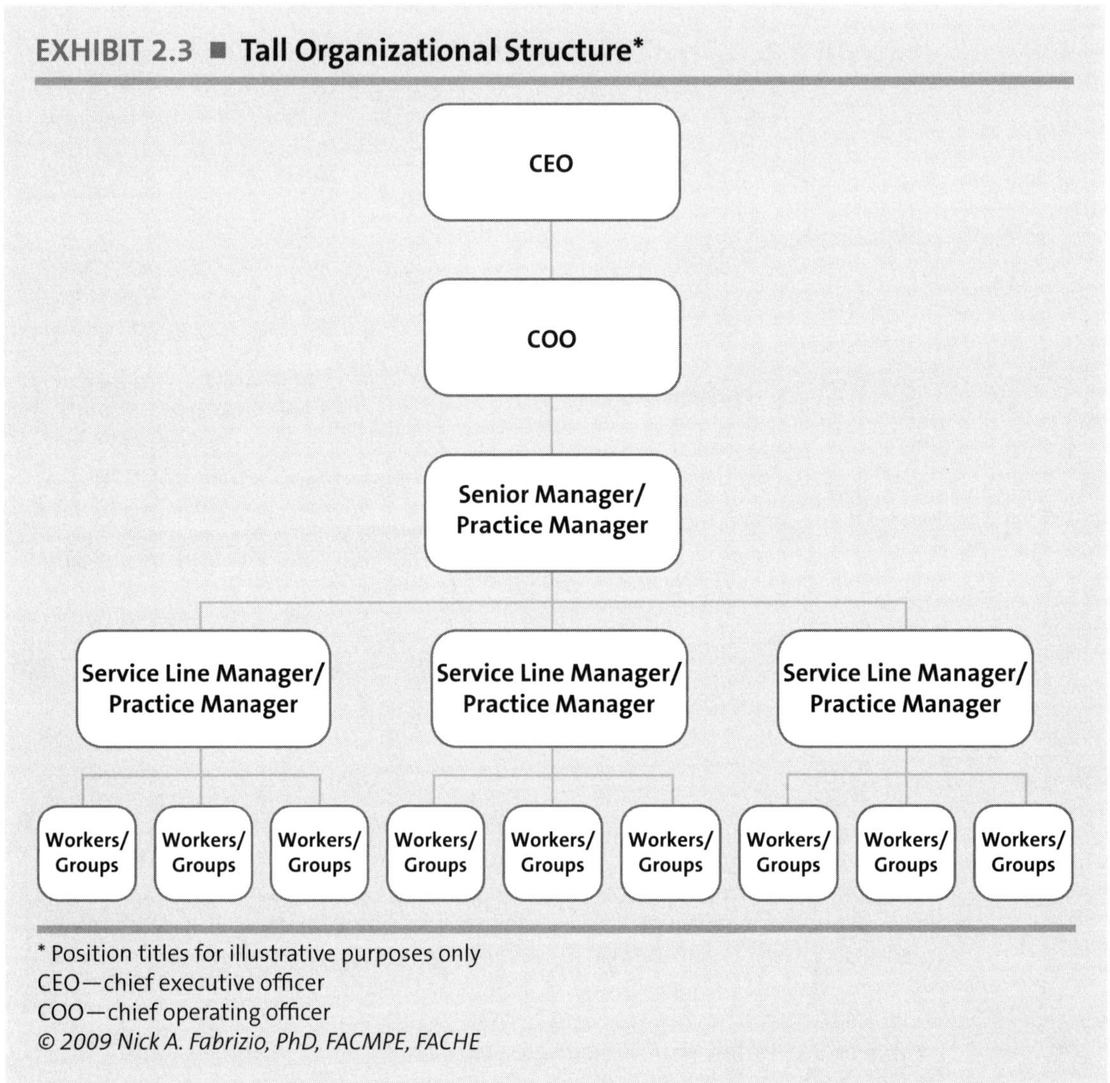

* Position titles for illustrative purposes only
CEO—chief executive officer
COO—chief operating officer
© 2009 Nick A. Fabrizio, PhD, FACMPE, FACHE

employees and providers in those practices and the CEO. These managers must be skilled in understanding medical practice management.

In undergoing a review of a system's organizational structure several considerations must be addressed, including the current gaps in performance and expectations, the number of staff and physicians, and job functions. The IDS must also determine what level of supervision is needed to lead the organization through its current and future challenges. It is clear that there is not a one-size-fits-all strategy to organizational design. It involves structured discussions with managers, administrators, staff, physicians, and board members.

In a *matrix* structure, shown in Exhibit 2.5, a manager has more than one supervisor. This is another organizational structure that is found in large health systems, including academic medical centers. In the matrix model, someone

EXHIBIT 2.4 ■ Flat Organizational Structure*

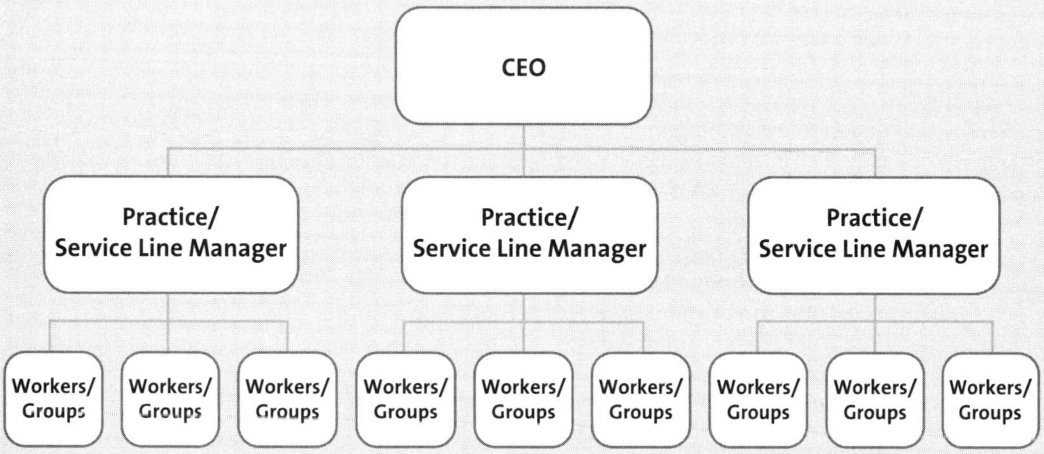
CEO
Practice/ Service Line Manager
Practice/ Service Line Manager
Practice/ Service Line Manager
Workers/ Groups
Workers/ Groups
Workers/ Groups
Workers/ Groups
Workers/ Groups
Workers/ Groups
Workers/ Groups
Workers/ Groups
Workers/ Groups

* Position titles for illustrative purposes only
CEO—chief executive officer
© 2009 Nick A. Fabrizio, PhD, FACMPE, FACHE

EXHIBIT 2.5 ■ Matrix Structure

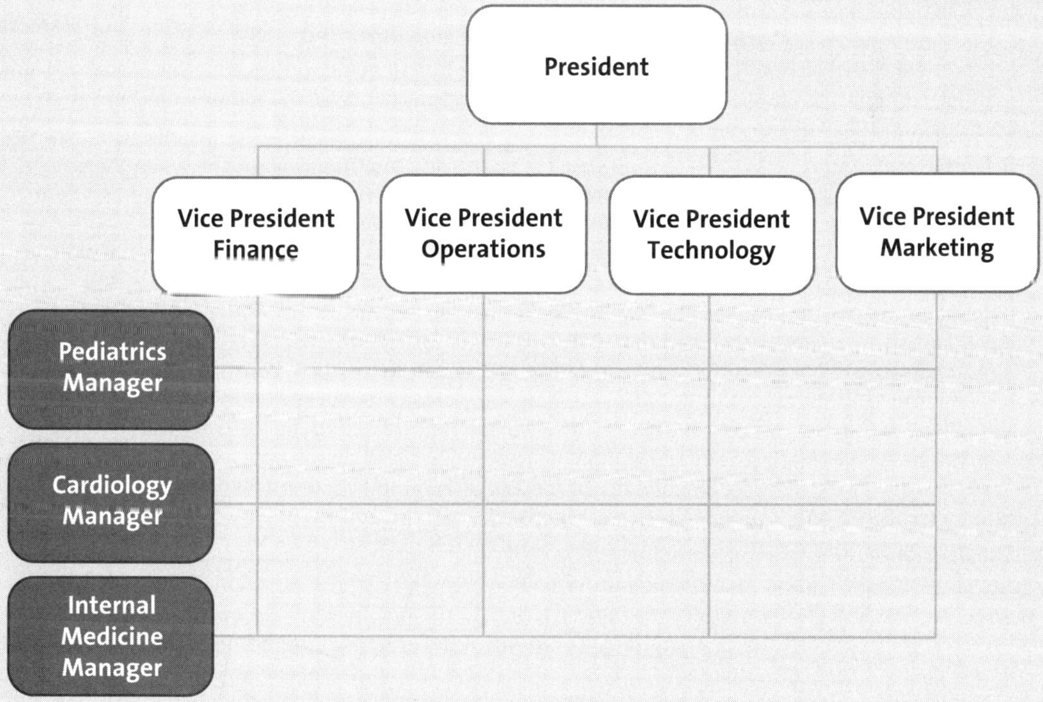
President
Vice President Finance
Vice President Operations
Vice President Technology
Vice President Marketing
Pediatrics Manager
Cardiology Manager
Internal Medicine Manager

© 2009 Nick A. Fabrizio, PhD, FACMPE, FACHE

▪ CASE STUDY ▪

Organizational Redesign of Kilkenny Health Care

Problem. The Kilkenny Multispecialty Practice (KMP) was part of an IDS that decided to undergo a focused review of its current organizational structure. Kilkenny was created in the early 1990s and started as a small internal medicine practice that grew to employ several different specialties and providers. Over time, the local hospital purchased several practices, including the KMP. Kilkenny multispecialty practice is now made up of more than 50 physicians from several specialties.

Unfortunately, despite its growth, KMP has done little to change its organizational structure. All of the physicians report to the hospital's vice president of medical affairs while all of the practice's office staff report to a hospital-based service line administrator who is filling two roles: one as the hospital service line administrator and the other as director of the hospital's several ambulatory care groups. Some of the complaints from the physicians in those groups have been that the organization is unresponsive to their needs by not having a clear strategic plan, not having a process to address their office operational concerns, being slow to respond to budget requests, and lacking clarity in its chain of command. The office staff of KMP did not know who their supervisor was and there was a disconnect between its clinical and non-clinical staff.

Study. The hospital leadership considered several organizational structures including a matrix form (Exhibit 2.6), which would have several people reporting to more than one manager. The hospital leadership concluded that this model was too complex and would be a more time-intensive structure to manage without a talented group of middle and senior managers in place.

Action. After careful discussions between the hospital and the physicians of the KMP, the hospital determined that a tall organizational structure (Exhibit 2.4) best met their needs. The structure provided clarity in that the hospital CEO was at the top of the chain (the system planned to have this function transitioned to a board over time) and it gave the physicians a medical practice leader who would work with them on compensation, quality, and practice concerns. It provided a full-time executive director who was responsible for the overall health of the practices including staffing, strategic planning, and budgeting. The tall structure also gave the medical practices their own operations, billing, and clinical leadership.

Outcome. While some may view the tall structure as having too many layers, the system was able to reduce staff in the information technology (IT) department, hospital finance, and general management so that it only increased the overall full-time equivalent (FTE) count by 1.5 FTEs of management. In analyzing the number of managers or layers, one must also factor in the costs of not having an adequate structure, which includes lost productivity, disenfranchised physicians and staff, and a failure to capitalize on the latest trends in technology and ancillary development. The plus side of the tall structure is that it provides more structure in having managers dedicated to the practices and an organized approach to handling current issues, including physician and staff recruitment and retention and future growth strategies. In addition, the operations of the medical groups are consolidated and report back to the executive director of medical groups. Similarly, the director of billing for the physician practices is a consolidated role that also reports to the executive director of medical groups. In this case, the operations, billing, human resources, and leadership are clearly defined.

The director of nursing in this structure works only with the medical groups, has a direct relationship with the system medical director, and works closely with the executive director. In this scenario, the clinic staff, including the nurses, report to their respective practice manager who then reports to the director of operations. This direct reporting structure is important to provide a clear chain of command. In practice, the director of operations works closely with the director of nursing for nursing-related matters to "manage" the nurses in much the same way as in the matrix design. The director of nursing is primarily used and consulted for training and development issues, quality improvement and performance improvement efforts, and developing policies and procedures.

who works in the cardiology division (clinic), for example, may report to both a cardiology manager and the hospital's vice president of operations. Advantages to this structure include having more expertise to a given area; fostering the development of cross-functional skills by employees and managers, which could promote greater teamwork; and potentially increasing employee involvement in management decisions or projects. Disadvantages include the potential for employees to be placed in the middle of turf battles between competing supervisors, lack of commitment by one of the managers to some new projects, too much time devoted to meetings, and a blurring of the chain of command, which may cause frustration.

An integration progression model related to growth and maturity of the organizational design structure illustrated in Exhibit 2.3 can be seen in Exhibit 2.6, which illustrates the framework of a large system with more than 100 physicians in several specialties. Because the system in this structure became accustomed to being partners with physicians and grew in terms of the number of practices and physicians it affiliated with, it necessitated the establishment of a separate and dedicated vice president of medical groups (VPMG). The main reason for this was that the system medical director (seen in Exhibit 2.7) could no longer fulfill his duties to both the system and medical groups. In this case, the system medical director focused on his inpatient responsibilities and the VPMG was responsible for the medical practices and worked with the vice president of ambulatory care to manage the physician network. The VP of ambulatory care has a more clearly defined structure under her control in order to delineate various functions and grow as the organization expands. In this

EXHIBIT 2.6 ■ Large System with More Than 100 Physicians in Several Specialties

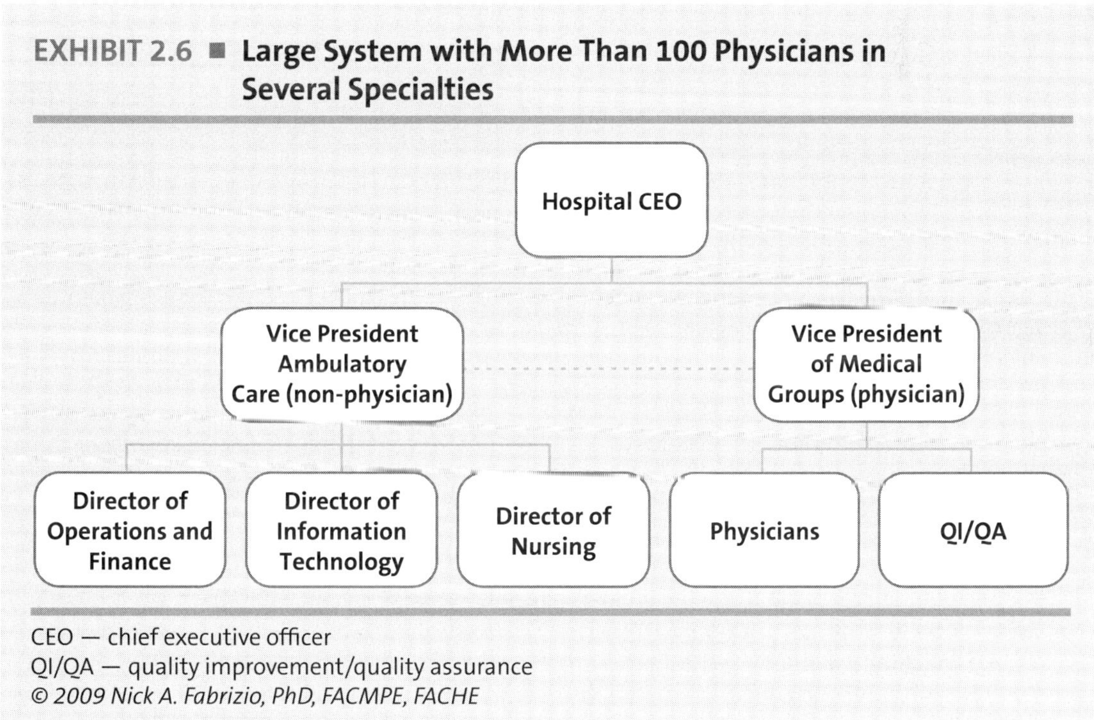

CEO — chief executive officer
QI/QA — quality improvement/quality assurance

EXHIBIT 2.7 ■ **Integrated System's Enhanced Structure**

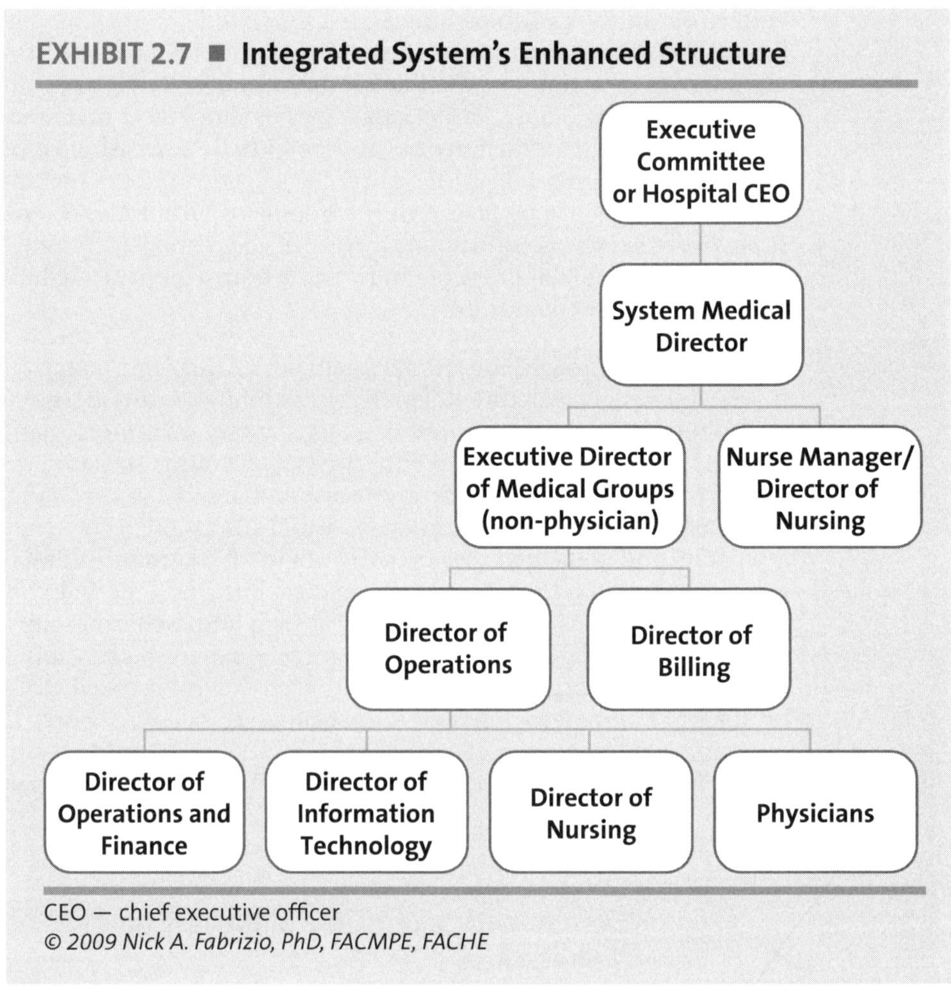

CEO — chief executive officer
© 2009 Nick A. Fabrizio, PhD, FACMPE, FACHE

example and in most cases, vice presidents of medical groups would devote 20 to 30 percent of their time to clinical activities (seeing patients) and 70 to 80 percent of their time to administration.

CONCLUSION

An IDS's legal and organizational structures, while interdependent, are frequently confused. The legal structure provides the foundational tools and relationships for the enterprise. A particular legal structure can certainly help to create opportunities and relationships that can facilitate or potentially hinder IDS goal achievement, but rarely if ever will legal structure determine whether the system will succeed or fail in achieving its goals.

On the other hand, the organizational, management, and supervisory structures of an IDS, along with individuals who work within that structure, provide the human framework and relationships within which the IDS will thrive, stagnate, succeed, or fail. There is not one perfect organizational structure for the IDS. Organizational structure varies depending on the size, scope, scale, mission, leadership experience, and leadership tolerance for designing and working within that structure. The organizational structure therefore includes the system's formal governance structure, including the management structure and relationships, committees within the system and its component parts, and the supervision and accountability structures within the organization. The organizational structure moves beyond the legal dimension to address governance, management and supervision, and relationships in furtherance of the IDS's mission and goals.

REFERENCE

1. D. Coddington, D. Moore, and E. Fisher, "Integrated Health Care Systems: The Key Characteristics," *Medical Group Management Journal* (November/December 1993): 76–80.

CHAPTER THREE

Legal Considerations for the Integrated Delivery System

Bruce A. Johnson, JD, MPA

Numerous laws and rules affect the organization and operation of today's integrated delivery system (IDS). These range from highly technical requirements associated with Medicare reimbursement, federal laws governing hospitals as tax-exempt organizations, state laws and rules dealing with physician and other service provider licensure and scope of practice, and dozens of other laws and rules including those governing employment relationships and state and local taxes. The range of potential legal issues and requirements that can affect an IDS's organization and operation is vast, and the application of those requirements to a particular system is highly fact-dependent.

Yet while the application of legal requirements to integrated systems is complex, certain key legal themes tend to affect the organization and operation of virtually all integrated systems. These include federal laws and rules that have uniform application across the United States such as the federal physician self-referral or Stark Law, the Medicare anti-kickback statute, and laws and rules governing hospitals and health systems as tax-exempt organizations. These legal themes also include various state-specific legal requirements governing physician licensure, the "corporate practice of medicine," fee splitting, and other laws and rules that combine to govern the organizational forms that may be used to employ or contract with physicians, and that may affect the terms of physician professional service relationships.

This chapter provides a pragmatic, high-level review of some of the principal federal and state legal issues that commonly apply to the organization and operation of integrated systems. Close attention must always be paid to the jurisdiction and fact-specific issues that affect the structure and operating format of an IDS in a particular community.

CONSIDERING THE CONTEXT OF LEGAL ISSUES

Legal issues tend to arise in connection with an integrated system's organization and operation, and in that context, specific legal requirements will affect how the system is structured and governed, how it delivers services, and its relationships with health care providers. To help understand the range of potential legal issues affecting integrated systems, we discuss the applicable issues by reference to the following organizing themes:

- The IDS's tax status and other characteristics as either a for-profit or not-for-profit enterprise;
- The IDS's legal structure and the nature of its relationships with individual physicians and other providers;
- The third-party payer reimbursement systems and strategies used by the IDS; and
- Legal issues that affect internal operations of the IDS.

Each of these themes is discussed in turn. Keep in mind that in addition to the issues discussed in this chapter, each IDS may also be affected by a host of other legal considerations, not to mention various business, political, and other considerations that will combine to create the context for a particular system's structure and operation in a particular community.

THE INTEGRATED SYSTEM'S TAX STATUS AND RELATED CHARACTERISTICS

A significant portion of the nation's hospitals and health care systems are tax-exempt, and various federal laws and rules governing tax-exempt organizations, including Internal Revenue Code (IRC) section 501(c)(3) and IRC section 4958 (governing "intermediate sanctions"), will have a major impact on the organization, operation, and arrangements within systems that involve tax-exempt entities.

Section 501(c)(3)

As a general matter, IRC section 501(c)(3) provides tax-exempt organizations special treatment under the federal Internal Revenue Code, provided that the organization engages in truly charitable activities such as the delivery of health care services. Tax-exempt status is generally available to hospitals, academic medical centers, and a host of other health care–related enterprises that engage in the delivery of health care services, provide medical education, and engage in similar activities.

Hospitals, integrated systems, and other organizations that seek and obtain tax-exempt status under IRC section 501(c)(3) are required to engage exclusively in charitable activities and ensure that the organization's resources do not "inure" to the benefit of private shareholders or individuals (commonly referred to as the prohibition on "private inurement"). Moreover, where the exempt organization must confer some benefit on individuals, that benefit must be conferred only incidentally and only in furtherance of the organization's charitable purposes (commonly referred to as the prohibition on "private benefit").

The precise application of these legal concepts to a particular organization or delivery system is situation- and fact-specific. However, as a general matter, tax-exempt organizations may engage in a wide variety of health care–related activities that are consistent with the organization's charitable purposes and involve "reasonable" compensation and other commercially reasonable terms. Thus, compensation arrangements under employment, professional service, or other relationships with physicians, individuals, and/or organizations as part of the IDS's business model must generally involve reasonable compensation that is consistent with the fair market value of the services. Notably, these standards are similar (although not precisely the same) to those imposed under other regulatory schemes including the federal Medicare program, the Stark Law, and anti-kickback statutes discussed in greater detail later in this chapter. Federal tax-exempt status is also typically a prerequisite for receipt of exemptions from state income, property, sales, and other taxes, although the precise treatment of such issues varies from state to state.

Intermediate sanctions

In addition to IRC section 501(c)(3), tax-exempt organizations are also subject to the requirements of IRC section 4958, which provides for the imposition of "intermediate sanctions." The intermediate sanctions law allows the Internal Revenue Service (IRS) to impose sanctions on certain persons who receive or approve excessive economic benefits from tax-exempt charities and social welfare organizations — including many hospitals, tax-exempt health clinics, educational institutions, and other organizations.

Where prohibited "excess benefit" transactions are found to have occurred, the intermediate sanctions law provides a remedy short of revoking an organization's tax-exempt status by allowing the IRS to impose penalty excise taxes on the individuals involved in such transactions. Such taxes may be imposed on persons who are influential to tax-exempt enterprises and either benefit from, or approve, transactions that are not consistent with fair market value. Specifically, IRC section 4958 provides for the imposition of personal excise taxes relative to excess benefit transactions involving certain "disqualified persons." Penalty excise taxes may also be imposed on the "organization managers" who approve such transactions.

As a general matter, an excess benefit transaction occurs when a tax-exempt organization provides an economic benefit to a "disqualified person" and receives less than the value of the benefit in return. Transactions that are consistent with fair market value will not constitute excess benefit transactions. For compensation arrangements, the law defines compensation to include all forms of cash and noncash compensation, including salaries, fees, deferred compensation, bonuses, severance payments, fringe benefits, insurance premiums, retirement plan contributions, and most other employee benefits, whether taxable or not, that are received by a disqualified person from the tax-exempt organization. Excess benefit transactions can also involve exchanges of property such as rent or loan arrangements between the organization and a disqualified person. They can result from both direct and indirect dealings between a tax-exempt organization and a disqualified person, including, for example, transactions involving intermediary entities such as a tax-exempt organization's taxable subsidiary.

Under the intermediate sanctions law and regulations, certain persons within the tax-exempt organization are automatically deemed to be "disqualified persons" who have substantial influence over the tax-exempt organization. Those include voting members of the governing body and persons holding a position comparable to that of president, chief executive officer (CEO), chief operating officer (COO), chief financial officers (CFO), or treasurer, as well as the organization's managers, such as the tax-exempt organization's directors, officers, trustees, and persons who have similar roles. Managers face potential double exposure under the law as they may be subject to penalty excise taxes if they benefit directly from an excess benefit transaction, and they can also be subject to penalties for their role in approving excess benefit transactions that benefit others.

For persons not falling into one of the categories referenced, a "facts and circumstances" test is used to determine whether the person has substantial influence over the exempt enterprise so as to be classified as a disqualified person. Factors that suggest substantial influence over the affairs of the exempt organization include when the person:

- Has compensation primarily based on activities of the organization that the person controls;
- Has or shares substantial budgetary authority, such as authority to determine a substantial portion of the organization's capital expenditures, operating budget, or employee compensation; and
- Has substantial management authority by managing a discrete segment of the organization that comprises a substantial portion of the activities, assets, income, or expenses of the organization as a whole.

The facts related to an individual's role, responsibility, and power within the tax-exempt organization, either individually or in combination, will contribute to a classification as a disqualified person under the facts and circumstances test. Department heads, certain key physicians, and other individuals within an IDS who are viewed as leaders in an important department, division, or subset of the organization are more likely to be considered disqualified persons — although the mere fact that a physician is involved in an IDS does not automatically make that physician a disqualified person for purposes of the law. Thus, while physicians who hold significant leadership positions in the IDS, such as serving on the system board or are physician executives, may be classified as disqualified persons, whether the intermediate sanctions law applies to these or other physicians who furnish services on the integrated system's behalf will depend on the specific facts and circumstances surrounding their position and role.

Disqualified persons who receive excess benefits are potentially subject to two levels of penalty excise taxes. The disqualified person must pay a tax equal to 25 percent of the amount in excess of fair market value, and if the transaction isn't corrected (by repaying the amount of the excess benefit plus interest before the IRS mails a deficiency notice), an additional penalty of 200 percent of the excess benefit is assessed. Tax-exempt organization managers who knowingly approve an excess benefit transaction can also be subject to a personal excise tax equal to 10 percent of the value of the excess benefit, not to exceed $10,000 per transaction. Accordingly, the law creates incentives for leadership in tax-exempt integrated systems to take steps and exercise due care to ensure that compensation and other arrangements are consistent with fair market value.

Intermediate sanctions and the rebuttable presumption

Among the steps and strategies that may be used to promote compliance with the intermediate sanctions law is the use of a "rebuttable presumption" process that, if followed, provides the benefit of a presumption that the transaction is fair and reasonable and not in violation of the law. The significant benefit of the rebuttable presumption process is if the transaction is later scrutinized, the IRS has the burden to prove the transaction was not consistent with fair market value.

Under the rebuttable presumption procedure, compensation payments and other transactions will be presumed to be reasonable if:

- The transaction is approved in advance by an authorized body with no conflict of interest in the transaction, such as by a board, committee, or other party authorized to approve transactions on the tax-exempt organization's behalf;
- That body (board, committee, or other party) obtained and relied upon "appropriate data as to comparability" *prior to* making its decision; and
- The board, committee, or other party adequately documented the basis for its decision concurrent with the determination.

Once the rebuttable presumption is established, the IRS has the burden to show that the transaction is not reasonable or is inconsistent with fair market value by demonstrating that the comparability data were unreliable or improper. Therefore, abiding by the process to establish the rebuttable presumption can be of substantial benefit to both managers *and* disqualified persons.

Other tax-exempt organization issues

Tax-exempt organizations are also subject to reporting requirements as consistent with the federal government's goals of promoting information transparency. Among the information reporting requirements are those contained on the IRS Form 990, the terms of which were significantly modified in 2007 to provide greater information transparency. Among other things, Form 990 reports provide information regarding the compensation level for key organizational managers and highly paid employees of tax-exempt enterprises.

An additional tax-exempt organization requirement relates to the restrictions imposed upon organizations that are the recipients of tax-exempt financing. Various covenants and agreements under tax-exempt bond instruments commonly impose restrictions on the operation and use of properties (facilities, building, and potentially other properties) used within the IDS. Tax-exempt organizations are also subject to the requirements of Revenue Ruling 97-13, which imposes restrictions on the use of tax-exempt bond-financed property and imposes requirements on management arrangements involved in certain structural models such as those involving management services and/or professional service arrangements that may be used as part of the IDS's business activities.

THE INTEGRATED SYSTEM'S STRUCTURE AND RELATIONSHIPS WITH PHYSICIANS AND OTHER PROVIDERS

The specific application of particular legal requirements varies depending upon the IDS's legal structure and its relationships with its participating physicians and other providers.

Basic legal structures

In Chapter 2 we reviewed a range of potential IDS legal structural models, including:

- Management services organization (MSO) models (involving a separate MSO that provides services to system-affiliated or independent physician practices);
- Hospital direct employment models;
- Captive subsidiary group practice models involving one or more physician practice legal entities organized as a captive subsidiary of a hospital; and
- Health system subsidiary models in which a hospital and physician organization are "brother/sister" organizations under a health system parent organization.

While these constitute some of the typical structural models, a particular integrated system is likely to involve other structures and relationships, and potentially a combination of several of these. Systems may also use other models such as the use of professional services arrangements in which physician-owned and operated practices will staff hospital-owned and operated clinics and/or hospital departments under contract. In this model, the physicians do not become hospital or health system employees, but the physicians and integrated system are closely aligned through the service arrangements, and the operation of the clinics or other facilities occurs under the IDS's overall governance, third-party contracting, and other arrangements.

The particular integrated system structure and the nature of its relationships with its physicians and other providers dictate the legal issues that will govern the relationships between the IDS and its providers for their services. As a general matter, the physician compensation arrangements will be subject to the requirements of the federal physician self-referral or Stark Law, laws and rules governing tax-exempt organizations (including the intermediate sanctions law and others), and other laws such as the federal anti-kickback statute. (Certain of these issues are addressed in more detail in Chapter 7, which concerns physician compensation.)

Various anti-fraud prohibitions are relevant to the organization and operation of integrated systems today. In addition to federal and state laws prohibiting false claims, such as the federal False Claims Act, and other laws prohibiting fraudulent activities, the federal anti-kickback and Stark laws, which are generally applicable to the federal Medicare, Medicaid, and other federal health care programs, are particularly relevant in the context of integrated systems.

Federal anti-kickback statute

Federal laws prohibit the payment of any "remuneration" for health care–related referrals payable by any federal health care program, including Medicare and Medicaid. Analogous state laws impose similar requirements.

The federal anti-kickback statute provides for the imposition of criminal penalties on anyone who knowingly and willfully offers, pays, solicits, or receives any "remuneration" — effectively, anything of value — in return for referring an individual to a person who furnishes or arranges to furnish an item or service for which payment may be made under Medicare, Medicaid, or other federal health care program. The remuneration cannot be made directly, indirectly, overtly or covertly, in case or in kind. The statute also includes any remuneration received in return for recommending the purchase, lease, order, or arrangement for any good, facility, service, or item for which payment may be made under Medicare, Medicaid, or other federal health care program.

Because of the anti-kickback law's potential breadth, it has possible application to a broad range of relatively common commercial activities in health care, including those involved in the organization and operation of an IDS. Because of this, Congress directed the United States Department of Health and Human Services, Office of Inspector General to promulgate "safe harbor" regulations that help to clarify the legal status of relatively common health care business relationships that may be relatively innocuous or even beneficial in nature but which might technically fall within the scope of the anti-kickback law's prohibitions. The safe harbor regulations specify a number of business arrangements that are afforded protection, or a "safe harbor," from the anti-kickback law's sanctions. In the context of an IDS, safe harbors that are often relied upon include those governing employment relationships, personal services and management contracts, rental of space and/or equipment, and others.

The Stark Law

In addition to the federal anti kickback statute, various legal and ethical pro scriptions prohibit or restrict referrals by physicians to entities in which the physician has a financial relationship. The most well-known such prohibition is the federal Stark Law, named after the law's chief sponsor, U.S. Representative Fortney (Pete) Stark. The Stark Law prohibits physician referrals of "designated health services" that are Medicare payable to entities with whom the referring physician or the physician's immediate family members have a financial relationship, *unless* the financial relationship falls within one of the law's numerous exceptions. The law defined financial relationships to include direct or indirect ownership or investment interests, compensation arrangements, or both. Designated health services include, among other things, Medicare-payable inpatient and outpatient hospital services, various forms of radiology and other imaging services, clinical laboratory services, and a host of other services that are furnished by physicians involved in an IDS.

Where a financial and referral exists, and those relationships do not comply with an applicable exception, the entity receiving the designated health service referral is prohibited from billing Medicare or Medicaid, the patient, or any third party for the services. In addition, any payment received in violation of the law's provisions must be refunded, and other sanctions (including civil monetary penalties and exclusion from participation in the Medicare program) can be imposed for Stark Law violations. Civil monetary penalties may also be assessed, including penalties imposed for each service provided in violation of the law. In recent years, alleged violations of the Stark Law have also been used by the government to "boot-strap" additional alleged False Claims Act, anti-kickback statute, and other legal violations.

Apart from the federal Stark Law, a growing number of state "mini-Stark" self-referral and anti-kickback prohibitions also exist. Such provisions may be reflected as more traditional proscriptions on fee splitting, which tend to prohibit much of the same conduct as the federal anti-kickback law, or they may consist of provisions that mirror the Stark Law in whole or in part at the state level. Many state prohibitions require disclosure of investment or financial interests, impose an outright prohibition on self-referrals as with Stark, or impose some other variation of the common theme.

Application of the anti-kickback statute and Stark Law to direct employment relationships

The nature of the contractual and legal relationship between the IDS and individual providers will have implications for the range of available compensation arrangements. For example, under the hospital direct employment relationship model, the Stark Law's bona fide employment exception is used to permit the hospital to pay the physician compensation for his or her services. This exception imposes specific restrictions relative to the payment and receipt of compensation. As a general matter, the employment exception requires that compensation must be based on each physician's personally performed services consistent with fair market value, and the compensation must be commercially reasonable.

Similar provisions under the federal anti-kickback statute govern compensation under bona fide employment arrangements. Common requirements under the Stark Law exception and applicable anti-kickback safe harbor include that compensation may not exceed fair market value for a physician's personally performed services, and that compensation must be commercially reasonable. In practical terms, this means that the hospital-employed physician may not receive production credit for services that are furnished incident to the physician's services, nor may the physician receive credit for work performed by anyone else. This restriction on how physician productivity may be measured may sometimes lead to a consideration of alternative structures involving subsidiary organizations within the IDS.

Captive and "group practice" models

In legal structures involving subsidiary models — including the hospital captive and/or health system subsidiary models — the subsidiary can potentially be organized and operated as a "group practice" under the Stark Law, and by doing so, additional opportunities and flexibility may be available related to physician compensation practices within the IDS. In any such subsidiary legal entity, the bona fide employment exception to the Stark Law may be used. However, the unique nature of a subsidiary legal entity is such that the captive subsidiary can potentially be organized and operated as a true group practice that can rely on the Stark Law's in-office ancillary services exception and that exception's more flexible approach to physician compensation.

An additional benefit of the use of the in-office ancillary services exception is that it permits designated health services that are furnished and billed by the group practice legal entity to be included and considered in legally appropriate ways in connection with the determination and payment of physician compensation. As described in Chapter 7, within a group practice that complies with the in-office ancillary services exception, measures of physician production can include incident-to services, and the overall pool of funds available for payment of subsidiary group physician compensation and other expenses can include funds from designated health services and other ancillary services furnished through the captive group practice. For integrated systems that are newly formed, this may sometimes be viewed to be of significant benefit as previously independent physician practice organizations become part of the IDS.

Nonetheless, in many integrated systems, financial concerns often lead to a realignment of the ownership of funds from ancillary services furnished within the system and its affiliated physician practices. Such a realignment may involve removal of ancillary services from physician clinics and relocation of such services to the hospital or a hospital-owned service provider. Alternatively, while many systems will retain the physical location of many ancillary services at a location that is in or adjacent to physician clinics in order to promote efficiency and patient convenience, the system may change the manner in which the ancillary services are billed (for example, from physician practice billing to hospital inpatient or outpatient clinic billing). This second approach, while often enhancing third-party reimbursement levels for the services, will shift the ownership of the ancillary service fees from the physician practice component to the hospital for financial management and accounting purposes.

Management service relationships

Apart from the mechanics of compensation systems involving employees within the IDS, other structural arrangements within the integrated system may also raise a number of legal issues under the Stark and anti-kickback laws. For example, where a hospital or health system operates a management services function that provides management, administrative, and other services to physician practices, the anti-kickback safe harbor governing personal services arrangements may be used, and where the Stark Law is implicated, the Stark Law exception for personal services and management contracts or another potential exception may be used. While the application of these requirements is highly fact-dependent, as a general matter these provisions require that the management services must be documented in writing, consistent with fair market value, commercially reasonable, and comply certain other terms.

Where a health system has a captive MSO that is truly independent of the hospital or the health system and is organized through the use of a subsidiary legal entity, the Stark Law is typically not implicated. On the other hand, some integrated systems operate MSOs as a department or division within the hospital, in which case the contractual relationship for MSO services may be with the hospital itself, thereby requiring compliance with the personal services exception or other Stark Law exceptions.

Other compensation-related issues

As noted earlier in this chapter, where a tax-exempt organization is involved in the IDS, laws and rules governing tax-exempt enterprises will also have implications for the compensation arrangements and terms within the IDS. The previously referenced requirements relative to section 501(c)(3) and section 4958 of the Internal Revenue Code, which provide for intermediate sanctions, also apply to the underlying compensation relationships. The combination of a tax-exempt organization, Stark Law, and anti-kickback requirements will, typically, require that the underlying compensation relationships with physicians and other providers within the IDS be consistent with fair market value and reasonable.

These same laws and rules also apply to service relationships involving physician practices that remain independent but enter into a professional services or similar agreement to staff a hospital outpatient clinic or otherwise work within an IDS. Under these models, the physicians typically reassign all or part of their fees for professional services to the IDS as permitted under Medicare rules governing reassignment under contractual arrangement, rather than pursuant to a direct employment relationship with a hospital or other component of the IDS.

In such professional service arrangements, the service agreement must be crafted to comply with an applicable Stark Law exception to include underlying contract terms that are consistent with fair market value, documented, and meet all other additional compliance requirements associated with the exception being relied upon. Such arrangements generally will also be crafted to fully or substantially comply with the personal services and management contract safe harbor under the anti-kickback statute. In tax-exempt organizations, because tax-exempt bond financing is frequently used in connection with the development of outpatient clinic facilities, personal service and management arrangements involving non-employed physicians are subject to the requirements of IRS Revenue Ruling 97-13, which imposes restrictions on the nature of compensation paid to physicians and others providing management services.

Employee benefits

The bulk of the discussion so far has focused on the character of the relationship involving physicians and an IDS as it relates to the determination of payment of compensation, but other laws and rules are also implicated by an IDS's structure and operating format. These include laws and rules under the federal Employee Retirement Income Security Act of 1974 (ERISA), which have significant implications for integrated systems and their benefit plans. ERISA was enacted to address many perceived problems in the nation's pension and employee benefit systems; all "employee benefit plans," including health plans and retirement programs, are within its regulatory scope.

ERISA is a complex statute with numerous applications that affect integrated systems in a number of ways. For example, ERISA has a direct impact on employee benefit programs including pension, profit-sharing and other "retirement plans," "cafeteria" plans, and others that can be offered by integrated systems as employers. Applicable ERISA rules impose a variety of requirements on such benefit programs that must be followed for the program and its underlying expenditures to receive favorable tax treatment.

ERISA also prohibits the establishment of retirement and other benefit programs that impermissibly discriminate in their benefit structure in favor of highly compensated employees through prohibitions on program participation, the benefits received, or on other grounds. Failure to comply with these applicable non-discrimination and related rules will undermine whether the benefit program is deemed "qualified" to permit funds contributed into the plan to receive favorable tax treatment. Non-qualification can have other implications for plan sponsors, benefit recipients, or potentially both.

Of particular note in the context of integrated systems is the application of rules contained in Section 414 of the Internal Revenue Code — the so-called affiliated service group rules — which require that in some cases employees of separate-but-related legal entities are considered to be employed by a single employer for benefit plan purposes. While the affiliated service group rules are complex and can have diverse applications, they are generally designed to address situations in which separate legal organizations work closely together, but seek to be treated separately for retirement and other benefit plan purposes.

Under the affiliated service group and related rules, two or more legal entities within an IDS are commonly treated as either affiliated service groups or under common control. In practical terms, the rules require that the welfare and/or retirement programs for these organizations must be cross-tested within one another to ensure that benefits do not discriminate against any subset within the organization. These rules apply in both tax-exempt and taxable (for-profit) integrated systems.

Integrated systems that are tax-exempt often use employee retirement programs under section 403(b) and section 457(b) and (f) of the Internal Revenue Code, or the IDS may establish and use a somewhat more familiar 401(k) benefit program. These systems typically provide a variety of health-related and other benefit programs. Experience suggests that while benefit programs within an IDS will differ from those available to physicians in private practice, the benefits are typically provided at a level that is somewhat comparable to, if not better than, what is available in many private practices. This fact, combined with the fact that the IDS is responsible for many of the benefit costs, while physicians as the owners of an independent private practice must pay these costs out of funds otherwise available for profits, typically make the actual dollar amounts available through benefit packages the same or better than those available in a physician-owned medical practice.

Other benefit concerns

Depending upon the legal structure and underlying state legal issues involved, other forms of employee benefits, most notably paid time off, which accrues and is paid over a period of time, may or may not be available in an IDS setting. Most hospitals have paid time off (PTO) arrangements to permit non-physician employees to accrue time off from work for which they receive separate compensation, with the total amount typically varying based upon years of seniority or years of service with the organization. Some hospitals and integrated systems elect to use this same PTO system with their physician and other professional employees, while other systems have determined that because the accrual of PTO varies from what is found in a typical private practice setting, the accrual of PTO to physicians is modified or eliminated.

THIRD-PARTY PAYER REIMBURSEMENT AND INTERNAL FUNDS FLOW

A third broad category in which legal issues arise relates to the integrated system's third-party reimbursement structure and format. Many integrated systems elect to use free-standing reimbursement systems, such as Medicare Part B, to bill for the professional services of the physicians and other non-physician employees. The actual reimbursement from Medicare is the same as that paid to a free-standing non-facility–based provider or a more traditional physician practice entity in that the Part B supplier receives reimbursement based upon the combination of the work, malpractice, and practice expense relative value units under the Medicare program. Under these models, the physician clinics are also treated as free-standing clinics and not as a department of a hospital. From a patient convenience and operational perspective, there is only one co-payment or deductible amount, and the payments for the services are provided by Medicare to the tax identification (ID) number assigned to the legal entity that owns and operates the clinic.

Provider-based reimbursement

The Medicare program also permits the use of facility or "provider-based" reimbursement for services furnished in certain clinical facility locations. Under provider-based reimbursement, two separate payments are provided by the Medicare program in connection with services furnished in a provider-based clinic. One payment is provided for the physician professional services, and the second is provided for the practice expense component associated with the delivery of services in a "facility-based" setting. The second facility-based payment is paid under Medicare Part A, and is only available when the clinic facility is operated as a hospital outpatient department. Some, but not all, states provide for provider-based reimbursement under their Medicaid programs.

Provider-based reimbursement is frequently viewed as advantageous to many integrated systems because the sum of the Medicare Part A and Part B (provider-based) reimbursement in at least some clinics is often greater than the Part B (non-facility) reimbursement available for the same services. As a result, for primary care clinics and certain specialty clinics, provider-based reimbursement may permit the IDS to optimize external reimbursement from Medicare (and in many states, the Medicaid program) for services furnished in certain physician practice settings.

However, provider-based reimbursement has its own limitations and associated costs including, most notably, the fact that patients are responsible for two co-payment and deductible amounts — one under Medicare Part A and the second under Medicare Part B. This may create inherent challenges within the patient population and at a minimum will require focused educational efforts to promote patient understanding. In addition, the use of provider-based reimbursement will affect the flow of funds within the IDS, and as such, will have implications for the perceived financial condition of the physician practices within the IDS. More precisely, because the reimbursement for facility-based professional services of physicians and other providers is reduced, and because the cost of practice overhead in the provider-based facility is paid to the hospital under Medicare Part A, this will have direct implications for financial statements and perceptions of the relative profitability (or losses) associated with the delivery of physician professional services and hospital outpatient services.

For example, under a captive subsidiary model that deploys physician employees of the subsidiary to staff a hospital-owned, provider-based clinic, services provided by physicians who work for the captive subsidiary will be reimbursed by Medicare in two parts. The Part B services will be paid to the tax ID number of the captive subsidiary at the reduced facility-based payment rate. However, the separate payment from Medicare Part A for the clinic overhead component will be paid to the hospital's tax ID number. The sum of the two payment methods — Part B (facility-based) plus Part A (facility-based) payments — are often greater than the Part B non-facility reimbursement. However, where provider-based reimbursement is used, the payment will be split between two tax ID numbers — the hospital's and the captive subsidiary's — which may affect the perceived financial performance of the captive subsidiary. While such internal financial issues related to funds flow and revenue attribution is important, in some integrated systems, they are not entirely recognized or understood.

The potential benefits of provider-based reimbursement must also be significant enough to outweigh the operational challenges associated with complying with provider-based requirements. Some of the challenges include the additional operational and compliance costs to ensure (1) appropriate oversight of clinical and financial operations by the hospital; (2) effective billing for provider-based services; and (3) appropriate cost allocation and reporting, including on the hospital cost reports. For example, all billing to all payers must denote an outpatient hospital service, even if the payer does not pay additionally for the outpatient facility charge. Moreover, the hospital must include the provider-based clinic as a location to which the Medicare three-day payment window applies, and the hospital's Medicare cost report must include all costs of the provider-based clinic in the same manner as other hospital departments. In addition, the hospital must meet each of the Medicare program's specific provider-based requirements, and establish a mechanism to ensure ongoing compliance. Provider-based locations will also be subject to requirements of the Joint Commission.

Commercial contracting

From a third-party contracting perspective, the IDS typically provides advantages in that the contracting power of the hospital and health system can be applied to physician services. Anti-trust laws and rules will apply to influence how various organizations involved in an integrated system can in fact be combined for payer contracting purposes.

Antitrust laws

Federal and state antitrust laws are designed to eliminate restraints of trade and related practices that restrain trade or interfere with competition. They are ultimately consumer and market oriented, and based on the policy rationale and premise that a vigorously competitive marketplace in a free market economy is good and valuable as a means to keep prices low and encourage efficient resource allocation, and will result in greater consumer choice of goods and services. Thus, under the policies expressed in antitrust laws practices and activities that undermine or hamper competition are viewed with disfavor. Numerous federal and state antitrust laws including the Sherman and Clayton Antitrust Acts, the Federal Trade Commission (FTC) Act at the federal level, and analogous state law provisions, affect health care business activities in every state.

Antitrust laws are likely to arise in the context of an IDS in two common situations. First, the laws may be implicated when the IDS becomes sufficiently large and powerful that it could be deemed to exercise "market power" within a particular marketplace. In general, market power is present when, because of its size in the relevant product and geographic markets, the venture has the power to control prices or exclude competition in a particular market.

In addition, while many integrated systems use direct employment and similar models with their closely affiliated providers, some systems also create other relationships with a broader network of physicians and other health care providers by establishing and operating network organizations such as independent practice associations (IPAs), physician–hospital organizations (PHOs), clinically integrated networks, and others. These organizations may raise antitrust concerns associated with "restraints of trade" that generally involve the "joint action" of two or more parties. Portions of the federal Sherman Act prohibit contracts, combinations, and conspiracies in restraint of trade. For a violation to be found, two basic requirements must be present: (1) there must be some form of joint action between two or more parties in the form of a contract, combination, or conspiracy (and not by a single entity), and (2) that joint action must be in restraint of trade.

In the context of integrated systems, concerns about prohibited joint action are usually minimized when the IDS involves only a single legal entity (such as a hospital employing individual physicians), or closely related entities as part of a single delivery system (such as a hospital and physician group that are captive subsidiaries to a health system parent organization). However, potential joint-action issues are more likely to be implicated where otherwise separate competing organizations (hospital-affiliated and independent physician groups) join forces in the framework of a new organization or under the umbrella of the IDS for contracting and other purposes.

Historically, in IPAs, PHOs, and similar network organizations, the enterprise and its participating providers either used a "messenger model" to dialogue with payers, or they sought to become "economically integrated" by sharing risk (for example, through capitation, risk pool, or other similar contracting arrangements). When sufficient economic integration is present, the network organization has much greater legal freedom to determine prices and other business practices collectively without becoming an unlawful restraint of trade — even though the network might involve participants who are otherwise competitors.

Clinical integration

In addition to economic integration, many integrated systems are beginning to develop organizational structures that include hospital-employed and independent physicians on a common medical staff who are engaged collaboratively to deliver cost-effective, quality patient care. These organizations focus on becoming "clinically integrated," given that this arrangement has emerged as a valid structure (recognized by anti-trust authorities including the Federal Trade Commission) and credited for bringing together competing and otherwise unrelated providers for quality-focused payer contracting and other purposes without violating antitrust laws. As noted earlier, historically, competing providers could only engage in joint contracting activities by sharing financial risk — but a properly constructed clinical integration and quality-focused program is now recognized as a lawful mechanism for provider collaboration.

Where clinically integrated networks are developed, they often include participation by one or more hospitals and a diverse representation among each hospital's medical staff. They will also use an interoperable electronic health record (EHR) that serves as the data platform for quality and patient care initiatives, coupled with systems to access and assess claims data. The clinically integrated network will develop focused programs that are directed at quality and cost, including clinical protocol development, clinical best practices, and monitoring linked to evidence-based medicine. Genuine commitment to quality is demonstrated by network physicians, hospitals, and others in focusing on quality initiatives. Third-party payers also consider quality and outcomes measurements, in addition to price, in determining reimbursement for inpatient and outpatient health care services.

A number of regulatory, technological, and operational changes are converging to facilitate the development of clinically integrated network organizations and initiatives as part of integrated systems. These include the adoption of exceptions to the Stark Law pertaining to physician self-referral, and the expansion of safe harbors under the anti-kickback statute that allow hospitals to actively support the adoption of EHRs and associated technology. These exceptions permit hospitals and health systems to sponsor and pay a large portion of the costs associated with new technology that can serve as a clinically integrated network's central nervous system. Additional developments include an increase in the portion of funds devoted by public and private sector payers to quality and cost management in patient care services, such as the Medicare program's Physician Quality Reporting Initiative (PQRI) and similar pay-for-performance (P4P) initiatives by commercial payers.

Additional factors contributing to the use of clinically integrated networks include the federal government's somewhat increased tolerance of exceptions to the anti-kickback statute for gain-share and related payment incentive programs and recognition of the potential value of in incentive alignment along cost, quality, and other grounds. The Centers for Medicare & Medicaid Services (CMS) has proposed a new exception to the Stark Law that, if finalized, would permit new "shared savings" and "incentive payment" programs involving hospitals and physicians. The programs would effectively build on gain-share, cost management, and quality-focused programs, such as PQRI and P4P initiatives, that are emerging as part of the agency's strategy to help rein in health care costs.

Likewise, with the increasing focus on cost management and coordination of care related to cost and quality, evolving third-party reimbursement systems are also likely to be considered for use in an IDS context. CMS is also testing the use of bundle payments for hospital and physician services for certain inpatient episodes of care for cardiac and other services, with the objective of providing for a single payment method for both hospital and physician services in order to better align hospital and physician incentives to promote increased quality and efficiency. While the demonstration program is limited in its scope, it likely illustrates the types of creative payment mechanisms that may be used by Medicare commercial payers in the future.

LEGAL ISSUES AFFECTING INTERNAL OPERATIONS OF INTEGRATED SYSTEMS

"Governance" models

The last broad category of legal issues includes those that affect the internal operations of the IDS. These issues include the laws and rules that affect the integrated system's governance, such as the laws and rules under the Internal Revenue Code. These rules affect the potential composition of governing boards and the powers and responsibilities of the governing bodies.

Of significant importance is the application of such rules to the governing board of captive subsidiary organizations and the role of physicians in the organizations that comprise the IDS. One of the greatest challenges facing integrated systems today is to craft arrangements that promote compliance with laws and rules applicable to corporate governance but that also promote significant physician involvement and influence in the overall operations and strategic direction of the IDS and its physician practice component. These issues are explored in detail in chapters later in this book.

Fiduciary and other duties

Members of integrated system boards of directors are always subject to fiduciary duties and responsibilities under state corporate law and other applicable legal principles, including duties of care and loyalty. Board members also are subject to confidentiality and conflict-of-interest provisions, and some governing boards have become subject to the requirements of the Sarbanes-Oxley laws and rules. All of these have varying levels of application on boards of for-profit and not-for-profit enterprises that may comprise the IDS. From a governance perspective, these various laws and rules impose requirements on the types of decisions that can be made at the board level, and they also require interested parties — which typically include physicians who are subject to governing board decisions — to recuse themselves or not participate in certain conflict-of-interest transactions. These laws and rules, as well as more general ethical principles and guidelines, will influence both governing board composition and the manner in which the governing body does its work.

The Joint Commission

Other legal and quasi-legal rules and regulations also affect integrated system operations. By illustration, the requirements of the Joint Commission governing accreditation of health care organizations clearly apply to hospital-owned and operated clinics. One of the potential benefits of IDS models using captive subsidiary physician organizations is the potential ability to remove the physician clinics from Joint Commission compliance. As a general matter, an IDS must meet Joint Commission standards when employing the direct employment models, because the physician practices are clearly under hospital ownership.

Employment laws

All integrated systems are subject to federal and state employment laws and rules. Because the scale of the IDS is much larger than the typical physician private practice in terms of the number of employees and scope of services, the laws and rules that may not have applied to a particular physician practice in a private practice setting may apply once the practice becomes part of the IDS. The scale of the IDS may require close adherence to other laws and rules such as the Fair Labor Standards Act, which encompasses state laws and rules governing the payment of overtime and other work conditions for non-physician employees and others.

One benefit of participation in an IDS is the availability of dedicated human resource personnel and management staff to attend to the additional human resource requirements imposed upon physician practices by being a part of the IDS. The various human resource– and employment-related laws and rules may sometimes represent additional requirements that were not available or applicable outside of the IDS setting.

Other employment-related laws include those governing workplace safety concerns such as the Occupational Health and Safety Act, requirements of state workers' compensation laws, and analogous state law provisions governing working conditions and others. Anti-discrimination provisions including the federal civil rights acts, the Americans with Disabilities Act, and analogous state law provisions will also apply. Such laws typically affect an integrated system's employment practices, as well as the way in which the enterprise does business.

CONCLUSION

This chapter presented a broad-brush survey of some of the key legal considerations that affect integrated systems today. Because every IDS is local, the particular state laws and rules must always be reviewed in connection with understanding what rules will affect the integrated system's operations.

Various laws and rules will typically be viewed as barriers — if not an outright hindrance — to the effective operation of aspects of integrated systems. Laws and rules certainly impose requirements and limits on what can be done and by whom. However, the seasoned participant in an IDS will view these rules as "rules of the road" that must be considered and addressed as part of the delivery system's overall business model and compliance strategy. The journey itself may be different than IDS participants are used to in private practice or other settings. But on balance, while the rules may involve a detour and slight change in the historic practices, they rarely constitute a barrier to accomplishing the IDS's goals.

CHAPTER FOUR

Governance in the Integrated Delivery System

Nick A. Fabrizio, PhD, FACMPE, FACHE

ROLE OF GOVERNANCE

Having an effective governance structure with committed individuals is critical to the long-term success of an integrated delivery system (IDS). Many integrated systems struggle to establish and maintain an effective governance function that is based on sound corporate practices. Governance can be defined as the process of decision making whereby results are measured by what is implemented or not implemented.

Much of our impression of corporate governance comes from the for-profit world. The corporate world gives us countless examples of good and bad governance. In recent years, the news media have reported several notable cases of corporate greed, corruption, and accounting scandals at large for-profit corporations. Poor governance was often an element that made these companies vulnerable. Poor or weak governance can also leave an organization vulnerable to competitive pressures and changes in the market.

Many medical practices are set up as corporate entities and tend to take a casual approach to governance. In the health care industry, hospitals are much further along the road of effective governance principles — the majority of hospital boards have more clearly defined roles, duties, responsibilities, and committees than do medical groups or physician-owned integrated systems.

As illustrated in Exhibit 4.1, an effective governance process serves to mediate the extended networks of internal and external relationships within the IDS and between the IDS and the community.

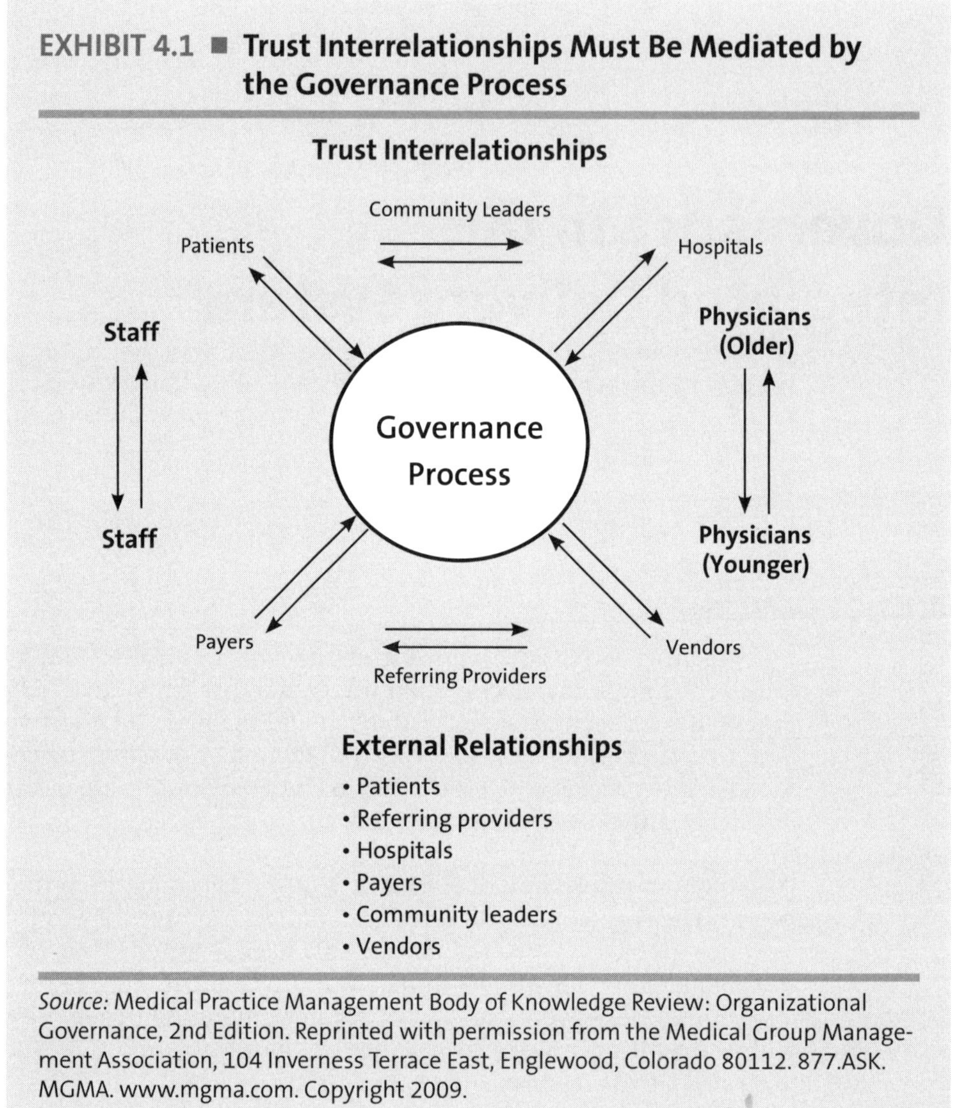

EXHIBIT 4.1 ■ Trust Interrelationships Must Be Mediated by the Governance Process

Source: Medical Practice Management Body of Knowledge Review: Organizational Governance, 2nd Edition. Reprinted with permission from the Medical Group Management Association, 104 Inverness Terrace East, Englewood, Colorado 80112. 877.ASK.MGMA. www.mgma.com. Copyright 2009.

DUTIES OF BOARD MEMBERS

Whether board members are paid or not paid for their service is determined by the IDS's legal entity. Board members in not-for-profit integrated systems are usually never paid for their service. Often, business and community leaders have seats on hospital or IDS boards. As a prerequisite for service, individuals serving on these community or selected boards should have an understanding of the health care field, the local economy, and the culture and climate of health care as it affects hospitals and physician practices. Clearly, having knowledge of only hospitals or only medical groups may limit the effectiveness of board members. This limited world view may also call into question whether prospective members can fulfill their fiduciary responsibilities as board members.

Board members must understand their fiduciary, legal, and ethical oversight responsibilities. The bar has been raised for all board directors after scandals in recent years at Enron, Adelphia, WorldCom, and other companies where board oversight was lax and board members were too compliant to management's wishes. As a board director, what questions should you ask management or outside experts? What level of expertise should you bring to an audit or a finance committee? What should shareholders, patients, doctors, and others expect from you as a director, and what should you expect from management? How can you ensure that the governance decisions you make are in the best interest of the organization? These are some of the questions that should shape board selection and service. Exhibit 4.2 explains in more detail the responsibilities and desired qualities of board members in a health care organization like an IDS.

GOOD GOVERNANCE: WHAT MAKES IT WORK

As illustrated by Exhibit 4.3, a good governing board has several important characteristics. These characteristics include being responsive, participatory, transparent, and willing to follow established rules. A good governing board is also accountable, effective, and efficient. The board must assure that there is a process to address conflicts of interest and that the voices within the organization are heard in data gathering and decision making.

Responsive

Good governance should allow for the input of all employees into the organization. For health care, this means that front-line employees — from the nurses to registration staff to the housekeeping staff — should have methods or processes for input into their jobs as well as the organization. This means that directors and supervisors must be team-oriented and solicit the input of their staff for the greater good. In this way, the board of directors will not be blindsided by matters that should be addressed by the organization's employed leadership. By allowing for greater participation and having a process where all staff has a voice in the organization, the board will have a better pulse on the organization.

Participatory

Participation needs to be informed, comprehensive, and organized. This means that in order to achieve the responsiveness mentioned earlier, workers, managers, executives, and board members must have the freedom to express themselves and be provided the forum to be heard. Having a culture and climate of trust and participation where individuals are allowed to express themselves and be heard without retribution will set the stage for open communication. This is easier said than done. Many scholars have written that it often takes at least four years to change the culture of an organization. Remember the adage, "culture eats strategy every day of the week."

EXHIBIT 4.2 ■ Sample Board Member Job Description

The ABC Medical Practice's Board Member

Job Description and Expectations

Purpose	To advise, govern, oversee policy and direction, and to assist with the leadership and general promotion of the practice so as to support the organization's mission and needs and to work closely with the administration of the practice in order to achieve its goals.
Number of Members	[Specify the number of members. The typical number is between 5 and 11, depending on the size of the group.]
Major Responsibilities	▪ Organizational leadership and advisement ▪ Organization of the executive committee officers and committees ▪ Formulation oversight of policies and procedures ▪ Financial management [to be defined] ▪ Review and adoption of budget for the organization; review of quarterly financial reports; assist administration with budgetary issues as necessary ▪ Oversight of program planning and evaluation ▪ Hiring, evaluation, and compensation of senior administrative staff ▪ Review of organizational and programmatic reports ▪ Promotion of the organization ▪ Strategic planning and implementation
Length of Term	[Specify length of term, which may be staggered.]
Meetings and Time	Commitment [Specify the time and location of meetings such as, "The executive committee will meet every other Friday commencing at 7:30 a.m., and meetings will typically last one (1) hour (this may need to be revised)." An alternative would be to have monthly meetings (2 to 3 hours) in the afternoon or evening (consider payment to participants).]
Expectation of Board Members	▪ Attend and participate in meetings on a regular basis and special events as possible. ▪ Participate in standing committees of the board and serve on ad hoc committees as necessary. ▪ Help communicate and promote mission and programs of the practice. ▪ Become familiar with the finances and resources of the practice as well as financial and resource needs. ▪ Understand the policies and procedures of the practice.
Board and Committee Structure	
Establishing Committees	It shall be the responsibility of the executive committee to establish ad hoc and permanent standing committees as necessary to assist in the functioning of the practice. Whenever possible, these committees should contain a representative of the executive committee to provide a proper liaison as well as an administrative staff person.
Typical Committees	[Include: finance, personnel, marketing, quality care, and technology. In areas where managed care risk contracting is a significant part of the business environment, a utilization management committee would be common to oversee the risk management of these contracts.]

Source: Medical Practice Management Body of Knowledge Review: Organizational Governance, 2nd Edition. Reprinted with permission from the Medical Group Management Association, 104 Inverness Terrace East, Englewood, Colorado 80112. 877.ASK.MGMA. www.mgma.com. Copyright 2009.

EXHIBIT 4.3 ■ Characteristics of Good Governance

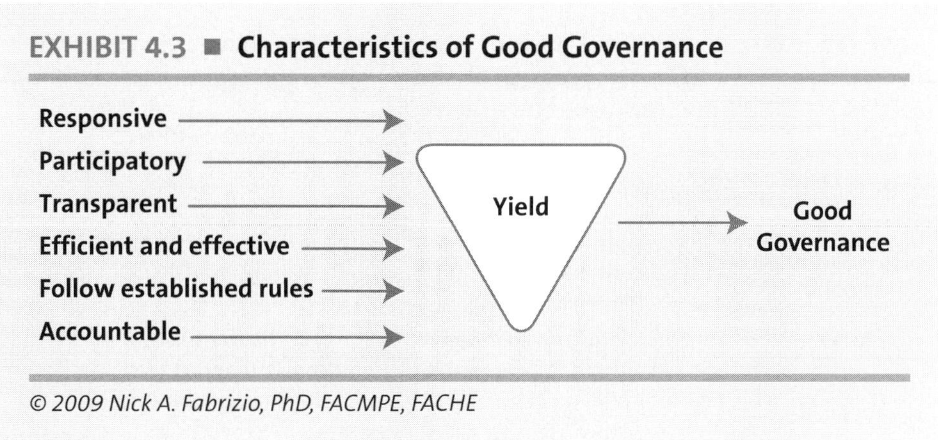

© 2009 Nick A. Fabrizio, PhD, FACMPE, FACHE

Transparent

Transparency means that decisions and decision making by the governing board of an organization are carried out in a manner that follows policies, procedures, and established rules. It means that the organization, employees, and physicians are free to exchange information directly and that information is accessible to those who will be affected by those decisions. Information that is distributed should be free from medical, legal, and financial jargon that limits the understanding and input from key constituents.

Organizations may also need to devote time to finding multiple methods to distribute information. There are several different ways individuals may hear and filter information. Some people like written communication that comes from standard print forms such as newsletters and staff bulletins while others prefer e-mail or departmental or organizational secure web sites. Still others prefer to listen to updates via traditional face-to-face meetings. The goals for leaders are to create multiple methods for getting information to the staff, physicians, and leaders.

Follow established rules

The organization must have policies and procedures that establish what its governance looks like and how it acts. The leadership team must have policies, procedures, organizational charts, and manuals that address how the organization is established, and where patients, employees, staff, physicians, and others go for help, direction, and to resolve grievances. Having rules may also decrease the number of misunderstandings that may result from how people perceive decisions are made or implemented. Having clearly defined rules may also help the organization's board members decide on the appropriate course of action.

Accountable

Organizational accountability is a key requirement of good governance. All institutions must be accountable to the community they represent. In health care, organizations must be accountable to several constituencies: patients, physicians, the greater community, the government, payers, and shareholders. An organization should be accountable to those who are affected by its decisions, actions, or procedures. Having a board that is responsible to the community it serves is of paramount importance. It is also important to note that without policies, procedures, and transparency, accountability is weakened and may not be enforceable.

Effective and efficient

Good governance should also ensure that the resources of the organization are used in the best manner possible. Organizations must be accountable to their internal and external constituents. Having efficient and effective processes that optimize the organization's resources should be a major management task. The board must ensure that its selected leader is in charge of developing processes that best utilize the community's most valuable resources — its people. The board must also ensure that the organization is acting responsibly in delivering health care and taking care of the environment.

ROLE OF THE CHIEF EXECUTIVE OFFICER

The role of the chief executive officer (CEO) depends on whether a business is organized as a corporation and whether it has a board of directors. In an IDS, the CEO's role may depend on whether the CEO of the IDS reports to the CEO of the health system or to a board of directors.

The CEO of an IDS is primarily responsible to carry out the strategic plans and policies as established by the board of directors. In cases in which the CEO reports to the board of directors, this person is responsible to set the direction, oversee the operations of the IDS, and ultimately be responsible for predetermined goals and benchmarks. In instances where the CEO of the IDS reports to a hospital or health system or to a physician council, the position becomes more complex and may have multiple power and reporting structures. The decision-making structure may act and react slower due to this dual or matrix reporting relationship.

Due to the delicate balance between hospitals and physician groups, the CEO in an IDS must take a strong leadership position within the organization. The CEO must be skillful in relating to both hospital administrators and clinicians. For this reason, the CEO must have credibility in both the inpatient and outpatient world. Failure to have these competencies or surround himself or herself with other key leaders who have these skills may marginalize the CEO's success. The CEO must also take charge of the IDS's strategy development and management systems, develop processes that collect and report information, and lead the board through the rapid pace of change in health care.

ROLE OF THE BOARD

The board of directors must have a clear strategy for charting the course of the organization. It must establish clear guidelines by setting responsibilities, and it should supervise and monitor the businesses of the system. The three legally mandated duties are centered on the concepts of care, obedience, and loyalty:

- **Care.** The board must care for the rights and needs of its members and ensure that the mission of the organization is followed. This includes exercising fiduciary responsibility. Meeting this standard requires that each board member must be knowledgeable of all information that is reasonably available and act with the appropriate care.
- **Obedience.** The board must follow the organization's bylaws and codes of ethics, as well as the common laws of society. The board must ensure that the organization is obedient to its purpose as described in its articles of incorporation and adhere to its mission.
- **Loyalty.** The board must manage its conflicts, carry out its duties unselfishly, and support all decisions made by the board (act as one voice) for the benefit of the institution and not to the board of directors personally. This standard also requires that board members *maintain confidentiality* in the decisions made when they are not to be a matter of public record.

The third criterion, loyalty, is most commonly called into question and is the hardest to manage. This duty is complicated when physicians or other community business leaders serve on the board that may have a stake in the health system's businesses, such as contractors, bankers, outpatient facilities, realtors, and attorneys. In order to facilitate this concern, board members must disclose situations in which they have a potential conflict, avoid competing with the organization, and refrain from discussing confidential board matters with others. Effective strategies to help mitigate these conflicts are to share meeting agendas in advance, actively engage board members during the meetings, and challenge them to review information and state conflicts prior to discussions related to those topics.

One of the most important roles for the board of directors is to select and evaluate the CEO. Other important and common activities of the board are to:

- Develop the organizational mission and vision statement;
- Hire, compensate, evaluate, and, when necessary, terminate the CEO;
- Establish criteria for providing quality care (the Joint Commission [1995] clearly states that the board is responsible for maintaining quality patient care);
- Monitor the organization and hold management accountable;
- Evaluate its own performance;
- Develop financial and other plans as appropriate; and
- Work with the CEO in monitoring goals and objectives.

Many organizations develop job descriptions to make sure prospective and current board members fully understand the roles and expectations of board membership. (Refer to Exhibit 4.3 earlier in this chapter for a sample board member job description.)

Board members must also understand their fiduciary, legal, and ethical oversight responsibilities. Clearly, given the recent problems in the United States' banking sector, directors are "on stage" every day through the actions of their

Questions Directors Must Ask

As a director, some of the questions you should keep at the forefront include:

- What type of questions should you ask management or outside experts?
- What level of expertise should you bring to a finance committee or compensation committee?
- What should the community expect from you as a director?
- What should you expect from management?
- How can you ensure that the governance decisions you make are best for the system?

organizations. Health care organizations must also address any potential for conflicts of interests if the board of directors includes physicians or even community business professionals.

Finally, the governing body must address the health care needs of the community by taking a careful approach to determining the number of specialty services the IDS provides, could support, and could afford by having (or not having) the desired number of physicians within those specialties. Unfortunately, not only is this problem complicated by supply and demand but also it is affected by geography, employment patterns, and the current health care needs within the community. Providers will want to know which medical services are already provided in the community. They also will want to know who their partners, covering physicians, or related specialties will be in order to transfer care efficiently, effectively, and safely.

HOW MANY BOARD MEMBERS?

In a recent survey of all not-for-profit acute care hospitals and health systems in the United States, including government-sponsored organizations, the Governance Institute found that the median size of the board of directors for all organizations surveyed was 12 members. The median number of medical staff physicians on those boards was two. In health systems, the board size reported was larger (median 16) and the number of medical staff physicians was again at two. The majority of these physician board members were reported to be on the medical staff but not employed by the organization.

In looking at meeting frequency, approximately 25 percent of the system boards meet 10 to 11 times per year with board meetings lasting 2 hours on average. Forty-nine of the 80 responding systems reported that the chief of staff was a voting board member in 39 percent of the institutions; 8 percent reported that the chief of staff was a non-voting member. One in four of the respondents indicated that the chief of staff does not attend board meetings.[1]

COMMITTEES

It should be the responsibility of the executive committee to establish permanent and ad hoc committees as needed in order to carry out the effective management of the IDS. Some of the typical committees that IDSs should establish include those that deal with finance, personnel, technology, quality, and compensation. Whenever possible, these committees should include a member of the executive committee as well as a physician (who does not have to be a board member).

Ensuring and improving safe and effective care should be a key consideration of IDS boards. Linking the hospitals and medical groups through technology and shared services should serve as the basis for improving the safe and effective delivery of care. The bridging of interests between their hospital and medical group leaders may be one of the primary reasons that IDS boards are more likely than hospital boards to have a committee that focuses primarily on quality (86 percent versus 58 percent).[2]

PHYSICIANS ON THE BOARD: RECENT TRENDS

Having physicians on the board of directors is one of the most contentious topics health care systems and hospitals face today. Clearly, arguments can be made for not having physicians on the board. These arguments include the overarching concern that physician involvement in board business presents an inherent conflict of interest for the physician. The main argument against this practice is that a hospital or health system will be making decisions, such as adding personnel (other physicians) or services (ancillaries), that physicians who serve on the board will not be able to discuss and/or vote on due to their conflicting roles in the health system. Unfortunately, this concern is often cited as the main reason to keep or remove physicians from board service. Instead, health system boards would be wise to conduct a careful review of board policies and procedures, the role of education, and a search for other appropriate options in order to gain the advantage of physician input into board business.

Other reasons cited for physicians not serving on the board is that the role of board members is to support the mission and maintain their institution's best interest rather than the physician constituency. This certainly places the physicians on the board in a difficult situation. Clearly, having other board members act as mentors to physician board members and providing continuing education about board responsibilities to these physicians may help mitigate this concern.

Another factor to consider in physicians serving on the board lies in the growing trend of employing physicians. Hospitals that have recently moved to a physician employment model attempt to integrate physicians into managing their offices or those service lines in an effort to have greater control over how those services are provided and marketed.[3] Clearly, if a health system employs physicians, the dynamics of the relationship between the health system and the physicians change. In light of this recent trend, boards in every community should debate the practice of employing physicians and having them serve on the board. A related factor that must be managed rests with the medical staff: they may view the employed physicians serving on the board as an extension of the administrative team and therefore feel they lack a truly independent physician perspective.

Another acceptable and creative way to bring physicians on the board of directors is to find retired physicians who are still in the community. Because these physicians are retired, they will not have the apparent conflicts that practicing (active) physicians may have. In addition, these physicians will likely be known and, as physicians, can help the board — and by relation, the IDS — establish greater credibility with the medical staff.

Given the complexities of managing and leading integrated systems, it seems clear that physicians will need to serve on boards to help bridge the gap in physician–hospital matters. Clearly, utilizing the strengths of administrators and physicians will give the IDS a competitive advantage. Physicians bring strategic, recruiting, and retention advantages to boards and their systems. In order for physicians to feel like true partners in strategy development and implementation, they must be part of the strategic development and management process. Physicians understand, relate to, and trust other physicians. This is important in order to understand the past, current, and future attitudes and beliefs of the medical staff, which also relates to recruitment and retention.

Another important consideration is that the most effective strategy for recruiting physicians is to have physicians involved in the recruiting process. Physicians can attract and sell the IDS to other physicians through the vast network of colleagues they have acquired through medical school, residency, and fellowships. This strong network of both physicians and residency/medical school program directors may help establish links and provide institutions with candidates that cannot be found by internal or external recruiters. Clearly, physicians should be leveraged for their unique and qualified perspectives.

An IDS must use the nominating committee to search for qualified board members, physicians included. The nominating committee must use explicit criteria and vet candidates based on their qualifications, fit, willingness to serve, and abilities to fulfill the duties of board service. The board must also have clear policies and procedures, which includes a board manual. This manual should be shared with potential candidates so that there is a mutual understanding of the time, care, and duties involved with board service. Another requirement is to have a clear conflicts-of-interest policy that is reviewed periodically by the board and during board meetings where potential conflicts may arise.

If IDS or health systems are truly interested in quality, they will realize the need for having physicians serve on the board. To achieve excellence, the IDS must have physicians on the board who are qualified and dedicated to putting the interests of the organization above their own. They must be focused on quality and providing a seamless coordination of care from the inpatient to outpatient settings or vice versa. Part of the success of improving quality lies in improving the management of information. Being able to share information to and from physician to physician and from physician to hospital will improve both the coordination and quality of care.

Clearly, in order to effectively transform health care, physicians and administrators of an integrated system must work together at the highest levels of their organizations. By working together, health care systems may avoid most of the current and past business deals that have centered on win–lose relationships. By having both parties at the table, the mutual goal of long-term, cost-efficient, and high-quality care can be provided. The ultimate goal is to provide safe, effective, efficient, timely, and valuable care to patients when they need that care.[4] Only when we meet these conditions will we satisfy the goals and desires of our external stakeholders including patients, insurers, and the government.

REFERENCES

1. The Governance Institute, *Boards x 4: Governance Structures and Practices* (San Diego, CA: The Governance Institute, 2007).

2. J. Jiang, C. Lockee, K. Bass, and I. Fraser, "Board Engagement in Quality: Findings of a Survey of Hospital and System Leaders," *Journal of Healthcare Management* 53(2) (2008): 121–135.

3. R.A. Berenson, T. Bodenheimer, and H.H. Pham, "Specialty-Service Lines: Salvos in the Medical Arms Race," *Health Affairs* 25 (2006): W31–W46.

4. M. Porter and E. Teisberg, "How Physicians Can Change the Future of Health Care," *JAMA* 297(10) (2007): 1103–1111.

CHAPTER FIVE

Organizational Dynamics and Culture

Nick A. Fabrizio, PhD, FACMPE, FACHE

People tend to blame the system or top management (or often, both) for changes that occur in the workplace. When groups or separate organizations come together to form a single entity or a group of entities under one umbrella, workers within those systems may fear that the changes will affect them directly. They also may worry that the changes will have a negative impact on their jobs. It is important to understand that change is inevitable; managers and leaders must create an environment in which communication is open and encouraged and where workers' concerns are addressed in a timely manner. By dealing effectively with change, leaders can reduce employees' stress over change and prevent it from rising to the point where they are calling the employee assistant program for help.

ORGANIZATIONAL CHANGE AND DEVELOPMENT

Because all staff and providers play such a key role in the delivery of health care, it is important for health care systems to have effective processes to understand, facilitate, and resolve issues related to change. Mergers, acquisitions, and alliances in all service-related industries and corporations in general produce anxiety based on what employees observe or hear. If not managed properly, this climate of change may produce uncertainty for workers, which can lead to issues related to lost productivity, absenteeism, workplace injuries, and even personal problems. Many large health care organizations have their own employee assistance program to help employees deal with their personal feelings about transitional issues or concerns.

Health care workers have a deep appreciation for caring for people and thus tend to have a deep attachment to their jobs. Their jobs, in part, define who they are as individuals. As a result, health care employees tend to have a deep commitment to the values of their organization; however, those values may not always match the organization's written values statement. It is important for leaders to know that they cannot change the organizational structure until they understand the current values of the organization, including those of its internal stakeholders — the physicians and employees.

Organizational development

Organizational development is the term commonly used in dealing with change in the workplace as a whole. The processes of organizational development, including the human and organizational factors, help determine how the organization predicts, responds to, and handles the changes in both the internal and external environments. One of the most important factors in managing change is how the organization meets the needs of its staff and other key internal stakeholders, who include the groups' physicians, administrators, and managers. Leaders must develop processes and systems that help the staff and other key internal stakeholders navigate through the change process. To help facilitate this change process, leaders can employ an assessment of the skills, abilities, attitudes, and performance of these key internal stakeholders.

Managing the changes

A challenge for an integrated delivery system (IDS) is to address how it will continually prepare for change. It is difficult in health care to enjoy periods of calm water for long. Even when the organization appears to be stable, changes are occurring. An IDS must continually look for ways to promote cooperation and information sharing and keep itself open and able to change.

Systems that facilitate change and adapt to change better than others are the ones that look for ways to promote change initiatives and then have processes to manage and lead those changes. The IDS must have a clear direction and determine how it will measure its success from both an organizational perspective and a human perspective. One organizational perspective might be to set a goal for successful integration of a key aspect of operations such as integrating a practice management system across all of its physician groups and hospitals. A human factor might be to set a goal for employee retention after the integration or merger.

To better manage the integration process, leaders must perform a mini SWOT (strengths, weaknesses, opportunities, and threats) analysis based on their assessment of the internal stakeholders' skills, abilities, attitudes, and performance. In creating the new organization, leaders must determine the skills of current employees and physicians by documenting any of those gaps. They must also determine what special abilities or competencies are needed to effect successful integration. They must carefully analyze the attitudes and beliefs of each IDS entity and what attitudes those entities will need to share in the combined or integrated model. Finally, leaders and managers must determine how the organization will measure and monitor the performance of internal stakeholders in order to successfully implement the new policies, procedures, training, and performance requirements to succeed in the new environment. The culture, mission, vision, values (CMVV) map, shown in Exhibit 5.1, helps illustrate the role of continual monitoring to deal with organizational change, improvement, and growth in the IDS.

Stage 1

As the organizations, hospitals, and medical groups come together, they bring with them their own cultures, missions, visions, and values. Some observers argue that regardless of where the IDS is in its life cycle or along the CMVV map, it must start at Stage 1 when new organizations are added to the IDS.

EXHIBIT 5.1 ■ CMVV Map

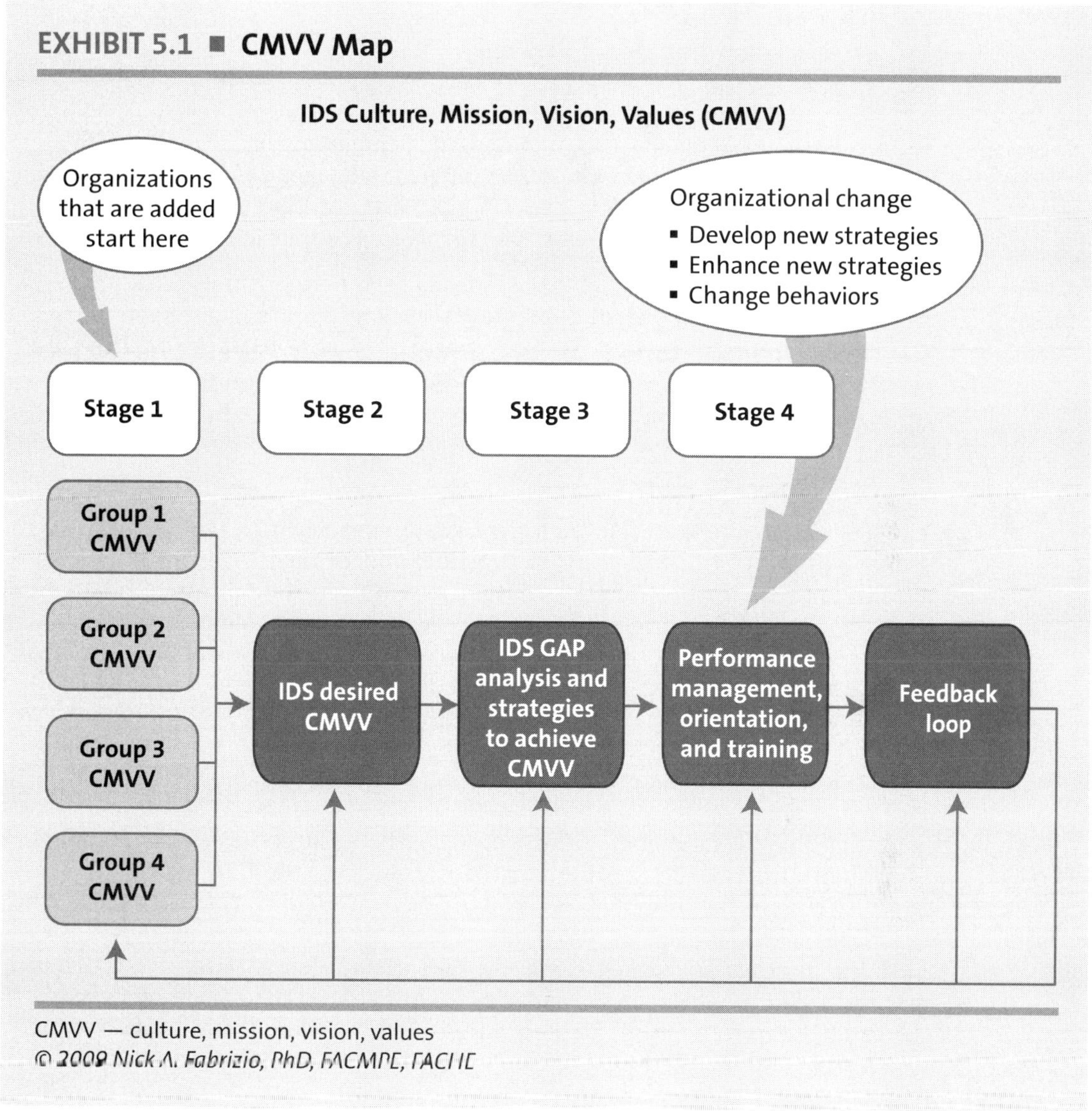

CMVV — culture, mission, vision, values

Stage 2

The leaders of the IDS must determine what the desired state is going to be. The leaders must create mission, vision, values, and beliefs principles for the new organization; these guiding and core principles will shape the culture of the entire IDS. This process should not be taken lightly as it often takes four to five years of dedicated effort to completely shape the existing cultures into one cohesive culture. This process is ongoing because the IDS will continue to add or subtract new members or groups, and the leaders will need to devote time to addressing the mission, vision, and values as a continuous process.

Stage 3

The leaders of the IDS must define the strategies that will bring the newly integrated medical group or other organization from its current mission, vision, and values to the desired state of integration with the larger organization.

The Cross-Functional Team Defined

A cross-functional team is a team comprised of employees and physicians from different levels of the organization with different job functions. For example, a team might be comprised of a physician, administrator, front-line manager, nurse, and a receptionist. This cross-functional team could address integration strategies, both opportunities or challenges.

The desired state will include the leaders working with other internal stakeholders of the IDS (the physicians, providers, managers, and staff) to: (1) solicit these stakeholders' input in recognizing where the organizations are now and (2) determine the strategies that will be needed and adopted to encompass the IDS mission, vision, and goals.

The IDS leadership must also perform a gap analysis, which will detail which groups or parts of the organization (hospital and/or medical groups) have specific areas to address. Some parts of the IDS will need to re-examine its mission and vision and determine how they can conform to and adapt to the IDS's mission and vision. At other times, the IDS leaders must look at an individual group's missions, visions, and values and determine whether they are a good fit with the larger organization, and how the IDS might be able to include any of the existing elements into the system's perspectives. This stage will involve a great deal of planning and time on behalf of the IDS leadership team and the individual medical group's leadership team. This is where a cross-functional team that includes members from various parts of the IDS can work together in a longitudinal fashion and report their progress to the IDS board.

Stage 4

This, the final phase of integration, dictates the implementation strategies to managers. The new processes that were identified and developed in the earlier stages will need to be implemented, monitored, measured, and evaluated by responsible and talented managers. The key to performance improvement is to develop detailed plans for how the organization, with all of its parts, will adhere to the agreed upon mission, vision, values, and goals and how these important organizational elements relate to system success.

Managers will be instrumental in taking the existing employees through a new orientation and training schedule so that the new expectations are clear and that current performance is measured, improved upon, or corrected throughout the stages shown on the CMVV map. As discussed earlier, because the IDS is not a static organization, when new groups are added or when existing groups leave, the system's leadership and the remaining groups' leaders must reassess where the organization is along the stages of integration and make course corrections.

FLEXIBLE PROCESSES AND CROSS-GROUP COLLABORATION

Groups and sub-groups of the IDS must come together to form cross-group collaborative teams. While in the later stages of integration these groups may come together spontaneously, leaders of an IDS in the earlier stages of development must create these teams and include representatives from the different parts of the IDS, including leaders from the different medical groups and hospitals. This combining of managers, physicians, and other leaders from across all groups may help foster a spirit of collaboration and working for the IDS. Forming these teams is a necessary but not sufficient condition for success.

IDS leaders must give each of these cross-group collaborative teams a charge or project to be responsible for. Each team must have a leader. The team members must have specific duties and expectations, such as participating in the meetings including attendance policies. The teams must be given a period of time they will be in existence and deadlines for completing assignments. The IDS board can lengthen the time these teams serve, but it is critical that they define as many of the ground rules as possible in advance.

The sub-groups or cross-functional teams of the IDS should have a method for collecting data and reporting results to higher authorities. Many medical groups within the IDS assign a senior executive to work with one or more of the sub-groups to ensure that they have top-level commitment and support. Those groups who receive information must in turn have a process for responding to that information, as these groups will help facilitate successful end-to-end processes that integrate technology, operations, marketing, and development.

The learning organization

To facilitate a changing environment, several theorists and scholars have promoted Peter Senge's model of the learning organization as a way to promote effective change. In Senge's book, *The Fifth Discipline*, organizations were described as places where people come together to continually expand their capacity to create results, be involved with the direction and outcomes of the organization, and continually evolve, work, and learn together.[1] The manufacturing industry has adopted this process successfully and more rapidly than other sectors.

Health care has been notoriously slow to adapt to change. One of the major breakdowns in health care in adopting learning organization principles is that physician practices and hospitals traditionally have not worked well together and there has not been a high level of trust between the two organizations. The other major limitation to adopting learning organization principles is that the physicians, their managers, and the staff often do not work well together as teams. The hierarchical model of health care — where the physician is at the top of the organizational structure and controls issues within medical groups, and where hospital administrators control issues within hospitals — must be broken down in order to effectively manage the organizational change process. These are clearly two important areas for improvement and a call for action for health care professionals.

Clearly, those organizations that have integrated physicians, administrators, and staff are better able to adapt to changes in market forces than others. Many also argue that in these team environments, the staff, which includes physicians, providers, and managers, works more effectively together and has a higher level of job satisfaction.

THE FIVE DISCIPLINES

In his book, *The Fifth Discipline,* Peter Senge describes five disciplines that help an organization achieve its purpose. The five disciplines are: (1) shared vision; (2) systems thinking; (3) personal mastery; (4) mental modeling; and (5) team learning. Turning these disciplines into strategies will help an IDS better integrate and adapt to a changing environment.

Shared vision

Shared vision is the discipline of getting everyone in the IDS on board with a common understanding of where the organization is going. Having a shared vision connects the IDS's ideas about what it wants to achieve with its people. A shared vision links the organization's vision with its workers and tries to align the corporate vision with individual visions.

To facilitate this learning, the organization must encourage its members to share their personal visions and help them connect their visions to the organization's vision. The systems leaders must create a safe environment in which they encourage their staff, which includes all of the groups' members, to share their ideas and help the organization develop a common set of goals.

Systems thinking

Systems thinking enables the organization to see how the individual parts relate to the whole. Systems thinking takes the individual groups' or subsystems' plans and enables them to relate to the IDS strategies. Each group must relate its success to the entire organization's success. This shift in outlook changes the playing field from small-group thinking to large, integrated, and coordinated efforts.

Another way to look at systems thinking is that the whole organization is greater than the sum of its separate parts. To think as a system, groups will have to change their orientation from making decisions solely in their own interest to thinking of how a decision will benefit the entire organization. An example of this is when a contract can be negotiated to provide advantageous terms to one medical group in the IDS but might hurt another group in the system. Instead, the entire organization must come to the table and negotiate as a system and leverage the size of the entire organization for the good of that particular group. While the outcome of this negotiation may not be as good for one group or entity as going at it alone might have provided, the resulting contract will be better for the entire system in the long run. It is important to remember, not only for that particular negotiation but also in training its members, that decision making must be done in the best interests of the system instead of a subset.

Personal mastery

Personal mastery refers to maximizing the individual learning that must be attained before organizational learning can occur. Leaders in an IDS must develop the skills to encourage participation among its members and an open dialogue among and between all of the different groups, hospitals, and employees. IDS leaders must orient and train system members to participate in a team-focused environment and also provide feedback to those members on the direction the system is going. To master this discipline, the organization and all of its members must understand the mission, vision, and values of the organization and see where they as members fit into the system and how they influence organizational goals.

Mental modeling

Mental modeling is the process of challenging the status quo and testing assumptions. It requires having a process in place for the internal stakeholders to form their thoughts, ideas, and strategies and having a process that enables them to test these assumptions with the system leaders to mold current and future strategies. One way a system can test mental models is to work with one of the medical groups that is implementing a service, such as extending clinic hours. The providers and managers in that clinic would develop a list of operational and clinical considerations that this initiative would have on patient care, current and future capabilities, and the quality-of-care implications. These considerations would give providers and managers a way to test their assumptions as well as measure the performance of the new venture.

Team learning

Team learning enables the organizational members to align their thinking about system issues with their individual group's issues and develop shared thinking and understanding. When parts of the system, or the groups, think about their issues in relation to system strategies, they learn to align their personal, professional, and group goals with system goals. Critical to successful team learning is the stated and observed attitudes of the system's leaders in encouraging and supporting team learning. If the leaders only pay lip service to team learning, the groups' members will quickly understand that this is more theory than practice and its success will be marginalized.

Team learning requires a culture and climate of trust and safety where individuals are free to express themselves in terms of their personal, individual work unit or group. They also must be able to address the IDS's strengths and weaknesses. To aid in the development of this discipline requires an open-mindedness by colleagues, managers, physicians, and IDS leaders. The goal is for each individual to learn from others, seek input from others, and search for alternative approaches to simple and complex work processes.

MANAGING THE CHANGE PROCESS: THE CHANGE AGENT

To successfully lead and manage the change process, there must be a defined leader or a small cadre of champions of change. These are the individuals who will lead the IDS in developing processes for implementing the change initiatives. Regardless of whether the IDS is in the early stages of formation or whether it is a mature organization and changing parts of its systems, it must have an identified *change agent*. The person who acts as the change agent and that person's activities may be different from stage to stage, depending on the scope of change and whether change is occurring across the entire system or just within a specific group or department.

Often the change agent will be one of the administrators or lead physicians from the IDS. This person will be responsible for organizing and coordinating the change initiatives. This person must take on the responsibility for developing the communication processes around the change initiatives, getting input from key stakeholders, creating project teams if appropriate, and communicating about the change process from top to bottom within the organization. This leader must identify support systems for people who struggle with implementing or adopting the change initiatives. This person will work with the IDS's human resources (HR) department and play an integral part in implementing the business plans and strategic plans. Change agents must continually communicate the objectives of the change initiatives and work with the board of directors or other senior managers on the project's status and must have the support of the board.

COPING WITH CHANGE

Leaders can help their organizations cope with change in a positive manner by taking the following actions:

- Identify the vision. Leaders must have a clearly defined vision of the change and be able to provide reasons for the change and discuss with employees what the end result will look like.
- Seek input. The more input people have in defining the changes the more they will adapt to and implement the changes.
- Embrace transparency. Employees of the integrating medical groups must know who their manager is and that this person has an open door policy to hear their concerns.
- Promote reasons for change. Successful change happens when each person understands why change is important and makes a personal commitment to implement the changes.
- Choose wisely. Managers from the group who are retained in the newly integrated organization (as well as any who are hired) must, in addition to their other skills, be great communicators and skilled in human resource management. Those who do not embrace communication will hold back the change process.
- Support employees. The IDS should make its central HR department available to all medical groups joining the IDS and ensure that these groups have the necessary skills and tools for the new employees.
- Combat negativity. Keep a flow of information coming to employees and physicians of the integrating group to help the new employees keep an open mind to the changes and be less predisposed to view the changes as negative events.
- Deal honestly. It is important that leaders always deliver the truth rather than the good news or the news that people want to hear.

- Extend help. Establish services, such as staff time, so that employees, staff, or providers can obtain help in dealing with change.
- Be patient. Give change a chance to work. It takes time to adapt to new environments.

CHANGING THE CULTURE

An organization's culture refers to its values, beliefs, business principles, traditions, ways of operating, and internal work environment. Organizational culture is developed in part based on these variables but also in how the organization:

- Defines its activities;
- Fosters communication;
- Establishes its values;
- Recruits new members;
- Strives for role clarity in defining employee job descriptions; and
- Ensures that its members are accountable for their actions and results.

Chrysler, General Motors, and Ford have long been trying to position themselves as more responsive to customers and agile in order to compete with foreign automakers.* More recently, they have been attempting to align themselves with combating the energy crisis. Chrysler's chief executive officer (CEO), Robert Nardelli, who took over as CEO in early 2007, has pledged to turn the company into a smaller and more flexible one. Chrysler and the other U.S. auto manufacturers have traditionally been large, corporate organizations with a traditional top-down management structure based on reacting only when it has compiled enough data in its hundreds of different divisions. Mr. Nardelli has vowed to change the culture at Chrysler by making it more responsive to customer and worker needs. He has scheduled "fireside-chats," which amount to evening meetings with his key executives, in an effort to empower them to lead their divisions and be more responsive to changing the organization.

Mr. Nardelli began thinking about changing the culture at Chrysler soon after he arrived. He noticed that some of the company's internal practices were centered around management promotions based solely on seniority rather than performance. He also noticed that sales forecasts were too optimistic, which led to poor planning and decision making.[2] Given that Chrysler is a large organization with hundreds of managers and divisions and thousands of employees, the change in culture there will take years and require a full-time effort. The jury is still out as to whether Chrysler can thrive as a business in the long term.

One of the main problems with changing culture is that it often takes three to five years to complete the change, which is a long time in the for-profit world unless the CEO has total board commitment. Having said that it takes "three to five years" does not mean that leaders should not attempt to change the culture

* *Note:* At the time of printing this book, rapid changes were taking place in the auto industry including the government's financial and organizational investment in GM and Chrysler. GM has closed several of its dealerships and is trying to reinvent itself as a leaner car company. Chrysler has exited bankruptcy and been bought by Italian car maker Fiat. The American auto industry is sure to continue to undergo significant changes throughout the next three to five years.

IDS Culture Killers

There are several factors an IDS should be aware of in leading and navigating through successful change initiatives. The following are among the attitudes to detect and address when implementing change-related activities:

- Changing because everyone else is changing;
- Holding on to what we are doing because it's the way we have always done it (The prescription for a slow but sure demise of the organization.);
- Not changing until we have enough data that prove we need to change (Also known as "paralysis by analysis," you may never get enough data to definitely rule in or rule out a change initiative.);
- Thinking that health care in your area is remarkably different than in other parts of the country;
- Waiting to speak with everyone about the issues before moving forward;
- Moving forward without getting enough input from key stakeholders;
- Not effectively communicating the change process;
- Not tying new initiatives to the system's strategies;
- Not developing criteria and metrics in advance to monitor the change initiatives;
- Not allocating the necessary resources, human and financial, into the initiatives; and
- Not providing the support structure for helping people cope with change.

of their organization; it simply means that leaders must have their board's commitment. It also means looking at ways to create short-term wins that the CEO and other managers can point to as milestones to changing the culture.

For example, in a large organization, it may be wise to focus first on how the change will impact the system as a whole. Then start the change process by taking one of the smaller, more manageable departments where there is strong leadership and fewer employees, and work on change initiatives there that can be measured and singled out as signs of progress. Citing these examples while working on changing the entire organization may help create and continue momentum for the leaders and staff of the IDS. These short-term wins may also prove to the board that progress is being made, which can help in the long-term effort to change the organization's culture. Refer to the sidebar, "IDS Culture Killers," for examples of behaviors that can set back culture and organizational change efforts.

BOARD INVOLVEMENT

The board can be both the CEO's greatest asset and greatest liability when working on change initiatives or changing the culture of the organization. As illustrated in the example cited in the previous section, it is critical for leadership to bring change down to smaller departments and show short-term improvements that can fuel longer-term initiatives. Clearly, the CEO must have board commitment when blending cultures or working on major change initiatives.

While it is important for the board to fulfill its fiduciary responsibilities, the CEO must find ways for the board to also be appropriately and adequately involved with the organization's culture without becoming overly involved. Leaders should think of ways, in advance, where board members can use their skills to serve as valuable resources for supporting the major change initiatives in the system. The following sections outline three guidelines that may help leaders leverage their IDS's board to get involved in and support the change process.

Gain board commitment

The board must be fully committed to the change initiative. Board members must show political support, which means they should express support for the CEO and senior management team. To nurture this support, the CEO must provide board members with the reasons for change, the status of the change initiatives, the names of those responsible for specific change initiatives, how many resources will be needed, and how the board will know when progress is being made. The CEO and other leaders should use this as their opportunity to explain to board members how they can support the organization's change efforts, both as individuals and as a board.

Provide tools to monitor progress

The board must ensure that initiatives have project plans and that implementation plans are clear; the board must be certain that the CEO has provided more than just a verbal report for how and why changes are needed. In order for changes to be successfully implemented, the board should expect to see how projects are defined, including the required human and financial resources along with a list of key milestones. This description might be in the form of strategic goals, initiatives, or work plans.

Leverage board members' skills

Board members provide many resources to an organization including their unique business, organizational, and other skills. The CEO or others in top leadership roles should determine how to involve (but not overly involve) board members in supporting change initiatives.

Board members may have technical knowledge or skills that will help the IDS make the transition to successfully introduce a new product line or service. For example, a board member may have expertise in developing an ambulatory surgery center or another type of free-standing health service site.

Board members may also have excellent planning and leadership skills that are well worth tapping into. For example, a board member from the community may run a business and know who in the community can help the IDS build a new facility. A board member who is a physician may have experience in productivity-based compensation plans who can work with the medical staff in considering alternative compensation models. A community board member may have extensive experience in fund-raising and could help develop strategies and processes for fund-raising to support special events or projects of the IDS.

When asking board members to serve on project teams, be certain to provide them with meeting minutes of their project team. While it may not be in the best interest of the change initiative to have board members involved with the operations of the system, there's no reason not to leverage each of their unique skills by assigning them to specific projects or strategic initiatives. The IDS board should also be involved with finding ways to address any strategic gaps that prevent the successful implementation of a new strategy.

FORM THE CEO–BOARD CHAIR TEAM

The CEO and the chair of the board of directors must be on the same page throughout the change process. Prior to bringing major cultural transformational initiatives to the board, the CEO should work with the board chair to educate him or her on the current state of affairs; the impact that current issues, procedures, or policies are having on the organization; why change is needed; and what will be needed to make things better.

It is important for the CEO to carefully assess the organization's SWOTs and identify a blueprint for how change will be led and managed. (A sample SWOT analysis is shown in Exhibit 5.2.) "Blueprint" is the key word, as many CEOs get into trouble by trying to specify too many details in the early stages of the change process. This leads them to make uninformed assumptions about when and how internal and external factors may change along the way. If CEOs get too specific in project plans or deliverables in the early stages of the change process, expect board members to remember those issues and hold the CEO responsible for sticking to that plan. It is more effective for the CEO to work with the board chair and help educate this person on the need to change and what support, mainly from the chair, will be needed along the way. Without the support and commitment from the board chair — stop right here!

Do an assessment

The board can help the CEO lead the change process by providing an objective assessment of the CEO's plans, issues, and results. While many leaders do not cherish bringing up problems to the board, these sessions should be viewed as an opportunity for the CEO to use the collective skills of the board to help move the IDS agenda forward. The board can often help the CEO frame issues in different ways that may be effective with different stakeholders. They may also offer new options to handle complex problems or opportunities. Think of involving the board in routinely assessing change initiatives by looking at goals in terms of short- and long-term timeframes and the effect these changes will have on the IDS and CEO's stated plans. This may help to avoid surprises and, perhaps the biggest danger of all for a CEO, losing the board's support.

EXHIBIT 5.2 ■ SWOT Analysis of Normalton IDS

Strengths
- Quality providers
- Extended hours that provide greater access for patients
- Improved utilization rates in the urgent care services delivered after hours

Opportunities
- Integrate EHRs in hospital and medical groups
- Create effective governance structure
- Expand services in growing community

Weaknesses
- Getting group consensus is time consuming
- Decision-making process is slow
- Outdated equipment and limited integration of EHRs throughout the IDS

Threats
- Competing hospital is adding physician services in the IDS's targeted community
- IDS is too slow to react to changing market forces

EHR—electronic health record

Educate board members about change

Board members tend to be results-oriented in their approach to board service. Therefore, take time to educate the board about why change is important and that it requires time, energy, resources, and strong leadership. The board is a part of this leadership. Consider filling board members' educational gaps about organizational management and change strategies by finding articles for them to read and bringing in outside experts to speak at board meetings on selected topics.

Evaluate success of change initiatives

The board should be involved in evaluating change initiatives. It is important for the system's leadership team to frame change initiatives into short- and long-term objectives and strategies so that the board can see immediate results and can follow longer-range projects. The board should be consulted with regularly, not just in financial statements but in operational and strategic change initiatives as well.

ORIENTATION, TRAINING, AND DEVELOPMENT

The IDS must focus its efforts on orientation, training, and development in order to successfully adapt to and lead change initiatives. Often training and development are two of the biggest weaknesses in an IDS and present the greatest opportunities for health care systems and medical groups to improve performance and change their cultures. Given that the dearth of training and development opportunities is such a problem in health care organizations of all sizes, it becomes a critical area in an IDS. Leaders must continually develop policies and processes that are focused on understanding the needs of its staff and the gaps and weaknesses of its medical groups and hospitals. With this understanding, the IDS can develop a systematic process to address those gaps. More important, this understanding enables the IDS to continually address orientation, training, and development in a systematic way.

Training and orientation is a continuous process because new employees enter hospitals and medical groups frequently. While the training and orientation of new employees slows the productivity of other employees in the short run, training and orientation are important. As the IDS adds new medical groups to its network, the employees, managers, and providers of those new groups must have a way to understand the culture, climate, and policies and procedures of the IDS. This requires a significant amount of time and resources on the part of the IDS. Given this commitment, it is hard to imagine that an IDS without an effective HR department can fulfill the requirements of sufficient training and orientation. Neglecting these important considerations may create tension and add to the shortcomings and limitations of true integration. These shortcomings may be borne out in a number of ways including higher staff turnover, failure to implement projects successfully, parts of the IDS not working well together, inefficiencies, and lower productivity.

Role of the human resources department in organizational development

Improving the training and development functions of the HR department is important to successfully managing and integrating multi-site departments. Also it is important to keep consistency and uniformity in HR resource policies to manage IDS staff in multiple locations. Another key ingredient to successfully integrating staff across multiple locations is to have individual departments or office managers work effectively with their supervisors in the system and with the HR department. Much of how the managers report and interact with one another is related to how the organization is structured.
(See Chapter 2 for more information about structuring the organization.)

The HR department should not be considered a stand-alone department. It should be integrated within the system by having one HR representative assigned to multiple offices/departments. That HR representative should interact with that department's leader and report to the hospital or system's leader (CEO, COO, or other senior executive position). The HR representatives should also have a forum where they interact with the providers, because the clinical and administrative processes need to be seamless across the system. Often this can be accomplished best by having members of the HR staff attend department or medical practice meetings. This coordination may help in achieving true integration and ensure that the need for consistency in the HR function is understood by all parts of the system. IDS orientation and training programs should be carefully monitored, updated, and stored on an electronic system that all employees and providers can access. New policy updates should be made available electronically, and all staff and providers within the IDS should have access to an HR intranet site where forms, policies, and updates can be easily updated, accessed, and downloaded.

One of the most challenging aspects of merging practices is that some providers in the various units integrating into the IDS may want to maintain their group's pre-integration salary and benefits program. While on the surface this may seem like a minor barrier, it may have legal implications and should be avoided at all costs. Doing so will not only create two or more salary and benefits programs, it will require separate policies and procedures and therefore increase the number of corporate or HR staff needed to manage the programs. While it may not appear at first to be a deal killer to integrating the new group to the IDS — and on the surface, you might think it's a small price to pay to capture a medical group — having multiple salary and benefits programs may kill successful long-term integration and possibly the IDS as a whole. It may create hard feelings from other IDS staff if they perceive that the salary and benefits program of another office is superior to their own. Even if the plan is cost-neutral, IDS leaders will not be able to defend the arrangement regardless of how many times they try. The system must maintain one common and consistent salary and benefits program that can be managed and implemented across all sites. Depending on the size and structure of the organization, it may be an option to consider to have these key HR functions professionally managed or outsourced in order to either save money or access superior expertise outside of the IDS.

CONCLUSION

As discussed in this chapter, there are numerous complexities related to organizational change that can impede the successful integration of different health care entities. Managing the change process by creating a collaborative and flexible organization that is nimble enough to adapt to and take advantage of the changing external environment is vital to integration and long-term success. The entire organization, including all of its parts, must be actively managed by its board and senior leaders as well as the HR department through a well-managed, structured, and collaborative process.

REFERENCES

1. P. Senge, *The Fifth Discipline: The Art & Practice of the Learning Organization* (New York: Currency Doubleday, 1990).
2. N. Boudette, "Nardelli Tries to Shift Chrysler's Culture," *Wall Street Journal* (June 18, 2008): B1–B2.

CHAPTER SIX

A Framework for Physician Involvement in the IDS Environment

W. David Holloway, MD, CPE, FAAFP, and Lisa Holloway, MA

Maybe it's useful for you to know who's writing the chapter you're about to read. I'm Dave Holloway, graduate of a 1982 medical class followed by a three-year residency in family practice. I opened my clinic and minor emergency center in a bedroom community close to a medium-sized city with a start-up loan from the hospital. In addition to trying to learn how to run a business — my practice — I found myself caught in the changing world of insurance reimbursement and contract negotiations. To try and get a handle managing the financial mess that was taking hours away from time with my patients and my family, I enrolled in one of the first executive MBA programs for physicians.

What I learned about business and leadership led me on a physician executive path that I did not expect to embark on but have found to be a most interesting journey in each of the three very different health systems I have been a part of. As my teenage son jokingly said after learning how to drive his stick-shift Nissan Sentra, "it's one sweet ride, babeeee!" The sweet ride has not come from finding a perfect program for physician involvement and then boiler-plating it in other organizations. Instead, it has come from learning the unique qualities and needs of each health care system and working to accomplish solutions appropriate to that setting.

Physician involvement matters deeply in the ultimate success of an integrated delivery system (IDS). I can't write a generic prescription for physician involvement, but what I can offer in this chapter is a brief insight into the physician's perspective and a framework to consider when looking at physician involvement.

THE DOCTOR WILL SEE YOU NOW

Because this is a chapter about physician involvement it seems right to begin with a reminder of just who we're involving. A quick look at how physicians come to be who they are seems like a good place to start.

I graduated from medical school over 25 years ago. My training ritual was a well-established tradition, and, though the arduous call schedule has been reduced to more humane hours, not much else has changed since then. Four key components were honed and embedded as I moved from medical student and matured into an experienced physician. They are worth noting because they affect how I as a clinician saw the world and how practicing physicians still do:

- I have to be in control to prevent bad things from happening. My patients can be harmed if I am not taking charge and watching everything.
- I want information assembled quickly. When I have patient history, test results, and the other data that I need in hand, I am a rapid-fire decision-maker.
- My patients look to me to tell them the best way to treat their illnesses, and because of this, my advising and advocacy skills are much better developed than my inquiry skills.
- Just like a plumber or electrician who gets paid by the project completed, our medical reimbursement system has made me quite comfortable with a piecework compensation program.

In addition, because of the years I spent developing medical expertise in my field, I expect respect for what I do, and I want autonomy in how I choose to do it. For years my hospital treated me like royalty and catered to most if not all of my whims. Of course I was content. Who wouldn't be a little giddy about respect, autonomy, and great cash flow? But now, my hospital is threatening to pull the rug out from under me. It is making pesky new demands resulting from external drivers such as quality and consistency. And then there are the patients who question best approaches for their care. So I guess the challenging conversation about quality, compensation, and control must begin, and I've never liked wearing a suit.

PHYSICIANS ARE PEOPLE, TOO

At every meeting of hospital administrators I attend, when the subject comes around to how to control the physicians (and it always does), someone remarks, "Trying to herd doctors is like trying to herd cats!" Then come the sympathetic chuckles. I'd like to point out that physicians are not cats. If you truly think they are then hire a collie to herd them and skip the rest of this chapter. Physicians are just like everyone else. Abraham Maslow did not exempt doctors from his Hierarchy of Needs — they, too, have a need to feel secure in the face of change; they want an income that makes them feel safe and successful, a job that makes them feel respected, and a collegial, friendly atmosphere to work in.

Like the rest of us, physicians are not necessarily excited by change, especially if they don't see the need for it and/or if they are excluded from meaningful involvement in crafting the change. Like the rest of us they must understand that the change they are going through will take them to a place that is better than the current state of affairs where the status quo is crumbling beneath them. Change-management experts caution that too often organizational leaders don't involve all the stakeholders who will be expected to support and implement the change. These leaders also do not spend enough time in exploration and dialogue about the current state and why a change might need to be made. Organizational leaders who skip steps in the change-management process and who exclude stakeholders such as physicians in decision making should not be surprised when those stakeholders refuse to buy into the change. Nor should they be surprised when these excluded stakeholders begin to display behaviors remarkably resembling those of an independent-minded feline.

CRAFTING THE FRAMEWORK FOR SUCCESSFUL INVOLVEMENT

Here's the money quiz. Seriously. Five questions. Don't cheat and look at the discussion below until you've given serious thought to your own organization in relation to these questions. If you're not willing to do that then you're not particularly interested in achieving true physician involvement.

Question One: What is your strategy for organizing as an IDS? Articulate your basic strategy in one complete sentence.

Question Two: How is your IDS physician group (IDSPG) structured for decision making and involvement? Where are the lines drawn for reporting? Briefly describe the IDSPG's relationship to your bigger organizational structure.

Question Three: Who manages and leads your IDSPG?

Question Four: What does the compensation plan for your physicians look like?

Question Five: How is the physician group considered financially in the IDS financial statements? Loss center? Investment? As a non-profit department similar to the executive teams?

The answers to these five questions will help you build the framework for physician involvement. So let's discuss what those answers tell you about the current state of physician involvement in your organization.

Answer to Question One: Strategy matters

Involvement begins with understanding what one is to be involved in. Constructive involvement of physicians starts with a clear strategy. It guides recruiting and location of physicians. It should guide physician and non-physician leaders as they make tough decisions about resource allocation. It will focus crucial conversations with the board of directors. Stephen Covey, author of the best selling *The Seven Habits of Highly Effective People*, tells us to begin with the end in mind.[1] This is great advice as a hospital thinks about physician practices. What's the burning issue that has caused you and your stakeholders to create, or think about creating, an IDS? IDS physician groups are tough. They are expensive. They are challenging. Why are you doing this? Hint: "Because everyone else is doing it" is not a good answer. Your strategic answer will provide focus for planning, governance, and recruiting efforts. A solid understanding of the strategy — the reasons for getting into this business — will prove valuable with the board and the physicians when the going gets tough. An institutional memory of the strategy will focus the inevitable debate and second-guessing that comes later.

Strategy is simply your unique approach to getting customers from a market. Many make it more complicated than it really needs to be. The steps are straightforward. Look at a market and find the desired segment, then look at the competition for that segment's business and craft an approach that is different and more compelling — better, in other words — than your competitor's. Get understanding and agreement, especially with the board. Then, translate the strategy into specific actions and execute.

At the core of any physician strategy is this: the health system's need to benefit from the unique relationship between a physician and a patient. The core transaction is that relationship. For the primary care physician, that transaction is most often a patient visit, leading to a health care decision. For the procedurally based specialists, the core transaction is a procedure. A brief strategic statement should explain what benefit is expected from owning these core transactions. (While my use of the word "own" might sound startling, I want to clearly differentiate "owning" from other ways to benefit from the core transaction, such as counting on, or hoping for a traditional relationship between the hospital and medical staff.)

Let's discuss the primary care physician strategy further. Why do you want to own primary care physician–patient visits? Write (or type) the answer beginning with "We need more employed PCPs because..." and then fill in the blank. Salem Hospital fills in the blank this way: "There aren't enough primary care physicians in our area to provide all the care needed for our community, and the private practices can't or won't recruit fast enough to fill the need. We will recruit and employ primary care physicians to fill needs not met by current physician practices." In a community where overall access to primary care is not a burning platform, a health system might fill the blank differently. For example, "If we don't own and operate our primary care network, our competitors will own and operate our primary care network. Visits to those primary care physicians will generate downstream activities for our competitors, not us. Not good." Salem's approach might be called an access strategy. The other example is a market share or network strategy. The execution activities driven by these two strategies will be different. For example, in the latter example, acquisition of existing practices is essential. But in Salem, acquisitions won't improve access, only new physicians will. Execution of these two strategies is different.

A specialty physician strategy will be very different from your primary care strategy. At the core of most specialty strategies will be the unique ability of the specialist to perform profitable procedures. Linking the primary care physician strategy to the specialist and hospital strategies is the final ingredient. This linkage is important down the road, when senior executives and the board are asking, "Why are our hospital and specialists doing so well financially, and our primary care practices are losing money?"

Ownership of the core transaction has an added potential benefit that can be combined with any strategy: alignment of quality incentives. Aaron Crane, chief financial officer for Salem Health, says it this way: "In the old world, physician incentives are not aligned with hospital incentives. This creates operational challenges and diverts management attention to independent physician agendas." Consider adding alignment around quality to your basic strategic statement. Salem Health offers an example of an access plus quality strategy. Because Salem Health recruits primary care physicians as an access strategy, selecting physicians who prefer teamwork and continuous improvement can smooth efforts to standardize around high quality, patient satisfaction, and reasonable costs.

Answer to Question Two: Reporting matters

On your organizational chart does your IDSPG sit at the same level as the hospital and report to a system-level executive team and then to a system-level board? And do physician leaders sit on the executive team and the system board? If so, you have created structure that will enhance physician involvement.

In 1994, Snapple Beverages was acquired by the Quaker Oats Company. Previously, Snapple had been outrageously successful. Brand recognition, growth in sales, profitability — all off the charts. Once in the Quaker portfolio, it didn't take long for the small company to lose the unique culture crucial to its success. Soon, the Snapple line of products was just another bottled ice tea. The *Harvard Business Review* observed that Snapple "went from local to national success and was poised to go international when the founders sold out to Quaker. The brand proved harder to manage than Quaker anticipated and in 1997 was sold for a fraction of its acquisition price."[2]

In a story remarkably like the hospitals that purchased and then sold physician practices in the 1990s, Quaker Oats Co. sold Snapple Beverage Corp. out of desperation for $300 million. This move came only 27 months after Quaker had spent $1.7 billion to acquire the maker of the trendy drinks. It doesn't take a number-cruncher to figure out that Quaker did not profit from the acquisition. On the contrary, Quaker lost $1.6 million for each day it owned Snapple. It's a common story line in *The Wall Street Journal*: a small, entrepreneurial company is acquired by a large enterprise. The larger company can't help itself. It imposes new forms, reporting structures, management style, corporate overhead, employee mandates, and quarterly financial targets, and soon the entrepreneurial spirit is lost in a sea of corporate requirements.

Hospitals are the most complex businesses on the planet. This is what business guru Peter Drucker found when he studied them. With all that complexity to manage, it's tempting for hospital leaders to think of adding physician practices to the mix as just another department. We already have an organization in place to run health care businesses, the thinking goes. Just have the new physician practices report into a manager who reports to the Vice President of Stuff. What hospitals will find, however, is that for all their expertise, hospitals and physician practices are completely different businesses. Just as Quaker Oats couldn't run Snapple as successfully as Snapple had run Snapple, hospitals find it much easier to maim a physician group than to run it.

Only once have I had a board member challenge the concept that physician practices and the hospital were different businesses. Earlier, I said the core transaction in a primary care physician practice was the office visit. The keys to the success of this core transaction are many: excellent scheduling, on-time patient flow, attention of a competent and caring physician, accurate coding of the visit for billing purposes, collection of the correct co-payment, and a dozen other small details repeated 20 to 30 times a day. Throughout the day, phones ring, prescriptions are authorized, copies of insurance cards are made, and exam table paper is changed. Bills are relatively simple and for small amounts. Often, the physician will personally review her accounts-receivable list regularly.

The hospital is far more complex and confusing. The core transaction is longitudinal care over days and requires hundreds of steps. Nurses are responsible for a multitude of tasks at the bedside. Patients are transported to far-away x-ray departments where expensive machines must be operated and maintained by experts. Medications are ordered from a central pharmacy and infused via intravenous lines, which are started and managed by other experts. The patients stay overnight in expensive rooms with electronic beds. The list goes on and on. Hospital bills are many pages long. Billing codes run in the thousands (compared to less than 100 most common codes in the physician office). And, there are so many different stakeholders that nothing is decided without a committee or two getting involved. Decision cycle time is long in the hospital, but this turns out to be unnecessarily long for most office decisions.

A mere mortal manager will not be able to run both of these businesses in parallel. Better to have a manager with a clinic mindset and playbook and another manager with a hospital mindset and a different playbook.

OK, we've made the case for creating a separate physician group, not embedding the physicians in the hospital machinery. How do we do this? While earlier in this book various legal and operating structures were discussed, the basic ways to link together physician groups and the hospital are the following:

- The physician group reports into the hospital;
- The physician group reports into the health system on the same level as the hospital; or
- The hospital reports into the physician group.

The latter option may emerge as the best practice in the future, as hospitals are seen more and more as just another cost center in a value chain. For now, in most markets, the second option makes sense for a number of reasons. Having the physician group report into the health system on the same level as the hospital recognizes the physician enterprise as different from the hospital and formalizes that recognition into day-to-day operations and governance. It is a concrete statement that says, with clarity, we are now a health system, not just a hospital with a lot of "non-core business units." IDS physicians need to see that their involvement makes a difference, and in this option, physician decision making does not get lost in the usual business of the hospital.

In thinking about physicians' involvement in the IDS, the fundamental question to ask is this: do we need a strong sense of ownership and responsibility from the people doing the core work of the organization? I believe the answer is "yes." We will very much need the physicians to feel ownership and responsibility for the challenges of quality, cost, and patient satisfaction. Don't push the physicians in your medical group down three layers in the hospital. The spirit of ownership you need will be crushed.

A key test is to view the physician enterprise from the board level. As a board member, do I govern as a health system or as a hospital? Physicians may resent governance that is stuck in the hospital world, but appreciate the balanced governance brought by a health system viewpoint. The physicians may not need nor want an independent board, as long as the health system board members govern the hospital and the physician group wisely to fulfill the overall mission (typically to serve the health care needs of a community).

With the physician group now seeing that the system organization is serious about its involvement, the leadership structure becomes important. Must-haves in leadership structure are:

- A physician-led committee with overall responsibility for the group;
- Physician-led subcommittees for quality, compensation, and recruiting; and
- A decision matrix, in writing, with three levels of decisions: those to be made by the physician group, those shared with the health system, and those made by the health system.

Examples of decisions that should require health system approval include the adoption of the physician group's business plan and operating budget, and launching joint ventures. Creating the group's business plan, while needing final approval from the health system board, is also a good example of a shared decision-making process. The plan would be drafted by the operations committee, approved by the health system board, and then executed by the operations committee.

Operations committee

I'll call the physician committee with responsibility for the group the operations committee. Other names are fine, such as the physician management committee or the physician leadership committee. Avoid words such as "governance" in naming this committee because there can be only one true governance body: the board of directors. Also avoid "council," which implies different tribes convening for building consensus, much like the medical staff organization. Limit the number of members; otherwise, the committee will be ineffective. Studies suggest between five and nine members for an effective team. A mix of elected and ex officio voting positions is common and seems to work well. For example, OMNI Medical Group in Tulsa, Oklahoma, has an operations committee of seven: an elected chair; physician-elected representatives from internal medicine, pediatrics, and family medicine (family medicine has two positions); a president of the group (a full-time employed position); and a committee member appointed by the system's chief executive officer (CEO). An odd number of members helps avoid tie votes, but in reality there will be very few split votes.

If the physician group within the IDS structure has been formed as a separate corporation, the written by-laws should spell out the composition and control of the operations committee. If the group is not set up as a separate corporation, it should still operate under the auspices of a document that has been crafted similar to a working set of by-laws.

Subcommittees

The detailed work of the operations committee will be done by subcommittees. The quality committee is tasked with developing a set of clinical quality metrics for the physicians (including patient satisfaction surveys), peer review, and process improvement initiatives. The compensation committee reviews the compensation plan throughout the year for compliance (with help of the IDS counsel or compliance officer). It also compares compensation to the marketplace and national surveys, and monitors the overall effectiveness of the plan. The recruiting committee is tasked with developing and executing an annual or multiyear recruitment plan. Each subcommittee presents recommendations to the full operations committee for approval. For example, the multiyear recruiting plan would be developed by the subcommittee, but final approval would come from the operations committee before any activity.

Physicians are more willing to be involved if they know their work isn't wasted. A key to avoiding wasted time and effort is to be as clear as possible in communication between the operations committee and its subcommittees. A best practice is to first develop a set of guiding principles and guidelines for the subcommittees. For example, if the group is committed to chronic disease management founded on evidence-based protocols, the recruiting subcommittee must know to include this as a must-have characteristic of any recruit.

Push involvement deep and wide

Systems entering into IDS structures are often confronted with the task of merging a number of smaller clinical groups and then having to determine how best to encourage constructive involvement across the sites. In 1996, Tulsa's St. John Health System chose to solve this problem in its physicians' group by creating a peer learning and involvement process for its 75 doctors called PPACTs (Patient and Physician Accountable Care Teams). Groups of five to nine physicians are teamed up (mostly by clinic or by combining small offices) to meet biweekly about medical matters such as testing and procedures and patient referrals that have been made between meetings. These discussions are often the catalyst for new office protocols and best practices.

In addition to reviewing medical matters, the teams are charged with reviewing clinic expenses, especially those generated by each physician. Comparing variable costs between physicians and offices produces ideas on ways to cut costs and operate more efficiently. The compensation plan includes a team component, based on overall utilization patterns for the local unit. Team behavior emerges through peer learning (and to some degree, yes, peer pressure). The team gravitates toward less variation from best practices. What a great way to respond to pay-for-performance plans in the marketplace.

The PPACT groups also serve as the vehicle for the operations committee to gather feedback when considering upcoming decisions. In addition, it creates an effective way to disseminate information to the physicians.

All physicians in the group are required to participate in a PPACT, and they receive compensation for doing so. Each PPACT group is led by a physician who is also a participating member of the group. The PPACT leaders meet monthly with the management team and receive additional compensation for serving as a group leader. As another side benefit, gathering the local leaders together frequently provides the perfect opportunity for leadership development.

Answer to Question Three: The management team matters

A well-run physician group produces results. By results, I mean bills going out and cash coming in, appointment slots getting filled, patients getting their needs met, and employees being hired, trained, and retained. Nothing will derail positive physician involvement faster than a poorly run business. However, just because the hospital side of the IDS business isn't well-equipped to get results in these areas for the physician group doesn't mean the physicians necessarily know how to do it either. Creating a top management team that pairs a physician leader with a great non-physician manager is the key to a well-run physician group.

The first pairing occurs at the top, with the physician leader of the group and the senior administrator. The physician leader should have a respected clinical background as well as a proven track record in leading physicians through challenges and change. This role will take significant time away from clinical work, so the group must pay a salary that compensates for expended time and energy, and the salary must recognize results. The physician role at the top should have the title of president or vice-president to indicate the importance of the position. The non-physician administrator half of the pair can have the title of director or executive director. This person often reports to the physician leader or the system leader.

The director must get results, or the physicians will insist on becoming involved in all sorts of areas where they don't belong day-to-day. Remember that control thing? Nothing will push the need-to-control button like an out-of-control accounts-receivable or chronic employee turnover. Hire an administrator with talent and a successful background in physician group management.

Repeat this structure on a smaller scale at each clinic site: pair a physician leader with a site manager. The site manager reports to the executive director and is accountable for results at the clinic site. The manager partners with the site medical director in ways that complement each other. For example, the manager is accountable for staffing the clinic and for making sure the patients flow smoothly. The medical director is accountable for working with the physicians on their appointment time management and appropriate use of resources. Great monthly results at the clinic sites will keep the physicians' need to control dialed way down, so they can see patients and put their energies for management involvement and oversight into working through the committee structure.

Answer to Question Four: Compensation matters

Compensation plans can influence physician involvement positively on three levels:

- Quality;
- Participation; and
- Skin in the game.

Quality

For most situations, linking a large part of physician compensation to managing patients will reward daily productivity. You are tapping into the familiar piece-work mentality most physicians understand and believe in. Each patient encounter is converted into work units (work RVUs) that are multiplied by a dollar amount. The work units capture the daily volume of patient visits in a standardized way. Chapter 7 discusses the details of various productivity compensation systems, but in terms of involvement, production is where you want about 85 percent or so of the physicians' attention and effort. Make the productivity portion of the compensation plan about 85 percent of the physicians' total pay.

Participation

If you base the entire physician paycheck on productivity, most physicians will not want to pull time away from their patient duties to get involved with running the group. Include participation in committee work and leadership as part of total pay. Doctors seem to be more willing to participate when they know that salary could be taken away for lack of participation rather than being paid an add-on bonus for committee and leadership work.

Skin in the game

Involvement in the long-term health of the entire enterprise can be encouraged by a system bonus of some sort. As long as the bonus is not directly tied to referral volume, the system bonus can reward physicians for their overall contribution to the health system. For example, in the St. John Health System discussed earlier in this chapter, the OMNI physicians could receive a system bonus if the entire health system outperformed the budget at the end of the year. The amount of money was not huge, but the message was important. I would avoid complex formulas; if the math is complex and for some reason the bonus is not paid, the physicians will be suspicious of financial manipulation. Keep it simple.

A few years ago Salem Health System initiated a new compensation requirement for its obstetrics hospitalists. Five percent of their salary is now tied to the requirement that each physician select, develop, and lead the implementation of one change initiative per year related to the improvement of patient care. After the physicians receive approval from the medical director for their initiative project ideas, they can request staff support such as project management and data analysis from other divisions in the system in order to complete their task. Response to this new requirement has been overwhelmingly positive, with great strides being made in patient safety and the patient experience.

Answer to Question Five: The financial statement matters

What do your board members' faces look like when they see the IDSPG line items on the monthly financial report? Looks of horror and dismay? Or looks of satisfaction that a major strategy is working?

Why is a chapter on physician involvement diving into financial statements and health system accounting practices? Let me fast-forward to the punch line:

it's hard to get meaningful involvement from demoralized people. Treating the physician division as an independent business unit with a freestanding profit and loss statement shows a lack of understanding of the physician strategy. It will result in looks of horror and dismay on the faces of your board members. It will demoralize your physician employees. The root of involvement, demoralization, and horrified looks is one and the same: failure of accounting to reflect the new reality.

My observation is that really smart business leaders on the hospital board of trustees and really smart hospital executives see the financial world through hospital lenses. Of course that makes sense; most people see the world through focused lenses. But, an IDS requires rethinking the entire enterprise. You have entered the world of the value chain.

All industries can be described as a value chain. From the idea for a product or service to acquiring raw materials, to crafting the widget for market to collecting payment, a chain of activities creates something step by step. Each step has a value, from tiny to great. A willing seller and a willing buyer determine the value in a free market. As your IDS gets into the primary care physician business, you will soon discover that the value placed on their services is low. The payment for their piecework as determined by Medicare and most third-party payers is much lower than payment for hospital or specialist services. And, the payments haven't kept up with the growing expenses of running a practice.

So, primary care physicians in private practice do what any business person would do under these conditions. They don't have expensive offices and furnishings. Often their employees don't receive market wages and benefits. They stop accepting patients covered by Medicare, one of the lowest payers. They seek relationships with businesses that need their services and are willing to pay more. A common example is a large multispecialty group practice, where the specialists cover more than their percentage of overhead expenses. In value chain terms, a group practice model places a higher value on the primary care physician than the piecework payment system does. The group causes value to shift towards the primary care ledger above and beyond what the third-party market pays.

For decades, the hospital has benefited from this arrangement. A large piece of the health care value chain was off their books. They received the needed product from the primary care physicians (patients) and services (that doctor thing they do), without the pain of the profit and loss. It's as if Toyota had independent auto workers show up everyday and build cars for Toyota to sell, but someone else paid the workers. Once the auto workers figured out they might have other options, the model would unravel.

The unraveling of this hospital-favorable model is exactly what we are seeing. At a time when demand for primary care services is rising, there are fewer medical students choosing family practice, pediatrics, and internal medicine. Primary care doctors completing residency have a plethora of options for employment at increasingly higher wages. Competition for a scarce resource has increased their value.

Yet, once the primary care physician is employed by a health system, the standard IDS profit and loss statement acts as if they are still in the piecework world. Payments for their services come in from third payers (yes, the same low payments that drove physicians out of private practice) and get posted to the monthly financial statement for the physician group. The expenses are subtracted (as both direct and indirect allocations, which can be mysteriously high in the hospital world), and — look of horror here — there's a loss.

The key to understanding this is to realize that you are no longer in the piece-work business, and to account for it in that way is delusional. As an owner of primary care practices you now own a new and expanded part of the value chain. Account for it as such. Actually, the hospital already knows how to do this. Look at your executive suite as an example. The outside world places no reimbursement value on the vice president division of the hospital. Your CFO wouldn't dream of sending a bill to someone for the executive team. Yet, it doesn't show a loss on the financial statement. The value is internal. The profit and loss for the overall business is designed to reflect this. No one pretends that the executive suite is an independent business. Likewise, the nursing division is not treated as a separate profit and loss center. Once you own the primary care part of the value chain, don't pretend it's an independent business anymore. This is a major mindset shift, but an essential one.

W. Edwards Deming, the legendary giant of systematic quality improvement, had as one of his seven deadly diseases: "Running a company on visible figures alone (counting the money)." He goes on to note that of course visible figures are important. "There is payroll to meet, vendors to pay, taxes to pay; amortization, pension funds, and contingency funds to meet. But he that would run his company on visible figures alone will in time have neither company nor figures." Deming advocates for an accurate understanding of overall value.[3]

Accurate reflection of the internal value has two huge benefits. First, each month the board and executive team don't get sidetracked in useless conversations about "red ink" in the physician practices. This is no more productive than if the board struggled with understanding the red ink in the executive suite or the nursing division. It pulls time and energy from the real issues around growth of the ancillaries and the service lines (which will grow if the primary care strategy is working). Second, it's demoralizing to the physicians to be labeled each month as red ink.

Of course performance is important, and the accounting should reflect actual performance. Rather than a simplistic profit and loss statement, use key performance indicators based on industry benchmarks. Chances are your nursing division in the hospital already does this. Rather than looking at their own profit and loss, the nursing division probably looks at key ratios such as patients per nurse. They look at nursing productive hours compared with volumes. They look at variance from budget. There's no reason to treat the physician division any differently. Another approach would be to allocate the physician division costs to the service lines benefiting from the strategy, such as lab and cardiology or orthopedics. Again, hospitals already know how to allocate costs to those profit centers that benefit from the IDS strategy. A third approach would be to recognize that most of the downstream revenue is generated by the physicians at some level (either through patient visits, referrals, or orders). All system revenue could accrue to the physician division, with all costs (read the hospital) also allocated to the medical group. The bottom line at the system level is what counts. If the physician strategy is soundly executed, the bottom line goes up. And physicians who see they are valued are likely to be enthusiastically, positively involved.

ONE MORE TIME

Growing up in Oklahoma, I witnessed more than a few oil-industry economic ups and downs. In the 1980s, I remember a bumper sticker saying, "PLEASE GOD, Just Give Me One More Oil Boom. I Promise Not to Blow It Next Time." Many hospital executives remember the last round of physician practice acquisitions in the 1990s. For many it was a bust. Consultants, Washington, D.C. think-tanks, and even Wall Street breathlessly hyped physician practice purchases by naïve hospital buyers. Hospitals paid too much. Ancillary revenue was moved to the hospital lab and x-ray departments. Costs went up. Income went down. Panic in the board room! And, in more than one market, practices re-privatized after big losses and unfulfilled promises. How'd *that* work out for you?

Physician involvement in the health system's strategy from the beginning is the key to getting it right this time. Slow down just enough to work through these questions:

- Can your executive team, trustees, and physician leaders all state your strategy?
- Is your group reporting at the health system level and do the physician-led committees cascade all the way to the front lines of the practices?
- Do you have top talent in the physician group management team?
- Does the physician compensation plan reward productivity, quality, and teamwork?
- Are you managing actual performance and achieving your strategy, or are you dead-set on the failed 1990s style profit and loss that would make Dr. Deming roll over in his grave?

The answers to these questions will determine whether you stand shoulder-to-shoulder with your physicians in an aligned and successful health system or become just another busy, confused, and scratched cat herder.

REFERENCES

1. S. Covey, *The Seven Habits of Highly Effective People*. (New York: Free Press, 1989).
2. http://harvardbusinessonline.hbsp.harvard.edu/b01/en/common/item_detail.jhtml?id=599126&_requestid=99652.
3. W.E. Deming, *Out of the Crisis* (Cambridge, MA: MIT Press, 1982): 121.

CHAPTER SEVEN

Physician Compensation in Integrated Delivery Systems

Bruce A. Johnson, JD, MPA, and Robert C. Bohlmann, FACMPE

An integrated delivery system's (IDS's) approach to physician compensation ranks as one of the most important factors affecting physician and IDS performance and success. This chapter reviews key issues related to effective physician compensation arrangements in integrated systems, including historical factors influencing current practices, features of effective compensation plans, examples of alternative plan methodologies, legal issues, and other compensation-related concerns.

In its most fundamental sense, an IDS's physician compensation program involves the financial model used to determine and pay compensation to physicians for their services. From an operational perspective, this requires attention to key financial issues including the attribution of revenues and expenses, as well as effective billing, collection, and financial management practices and systems within the IDS. Compensation plans also play an important role in shaping provider behavior by functioning as a critical component of the overall incentive and performance feedback system for the IDS physicians. Effective compensation practices are therefore essential to the IDS's success and to the professional success and satisfaction of the organization's physicians.

EFFECTIVE COMPENSATION PLANS: HISTORICAL DIMENSIONS AND PRESENT CONDITIONS

Experience shows that there is no single "best" approach to physician compensation in an IDS, just as there is no single approach that is perfectly "fair." Each compensation plan will be shaped by the IDS's particular mix of practice specialties, goals, values, culture, age and maturity, positive and negative experiences of the past, and other factors.

Current-day compensation methodologies in integrated systems should be distinguished from the systems that existed in the late 1980s through the mid-to-late 1990s. During this period the IDS learning curve was steep and, to a certain degree, not based on realistic financial and/or business principles. Integrated systems competed with physician practice management companies in the purchase and operation of medical practices. Because of the competitive nature of the environment, the practical business objectives of many integrated systems focused primarily on practice acquisition, leading to an almost "anything goes" approach to physician compensation. As a result, many of the compensation practices during this period were completely beyond reality in that they involved financial models and incentive systems that were not based on sound financial assumptions and practices, and therefore largely unsustainable.

The combination of huge financial losses and other factors that were present in many integrated systems formed in the 1990s commonly led to a re-evaluation and, frequently, the termination of physician employment arrangements. These changes were, in many instances, accomplished through complete IDS dissolution or "privatization" of IDS physician practices.

Yet many integrated systems — including those comprised of large systems — determined that the initial strategy involving bringing physicians, hospitals, and other aspects of the health care delivery system under a "big tent" was sound, but their approach to implementation (including implementation of physician compensation practices) was faulty. Many of these systems elected to re-engineer their physician relationships by changing their physician compensation plans and related relationship terms in order to develop more realistic relationships. These new relationships typically created a closer link between a physician's compensation and his or her work levels or production. They were also built on financial models that were more sustainable in the near and long term.

Overall, the compensation practices of the 1980s and 1990s in which physicians were paid large sums in connection with practice acquisition and largely fixed salaries over extended periods that resulted in large financial losses, were replaced by production-oriented, market competitive, and financially sustainable compensation practices. Remembering yesterday's failures is important in considering compensation practices for today's integrated systems. These lessons from the past will help IDS leaders to both understand the features of successful compensation practices and also help to refute efforts to reinstitute approaches that proved to be unrealistic and unsustainable in the past.

Past and more recent experiences suggest that while there is no single perfect or "right" compensation system for an IDS, effective compensation plans in an IDS tend to share a number of common features, including those discussed as follows.

Goal directed

Effective compensation practices are designed to promote and align the shared goals of the IDS and its physicians. Those goals tend to be multifaceted, but they will commonly include:

- Encouraging and rewarding production and work;
- Promoting cost management;

- Providing quality care;
- Enhancing patient and other "customer" satisfaction;
- Promoting physician "control" and "influence" over the compensation they will eventually receive; and
- Rewarding and teaching research, outreach, and other activities that are critical to the physician's clinical satisfaction and the practice's success.

Sustainable

Effective plans will tend to be sustainable in different ways. One form of sustainability relates to ensuring that the compensation system is compatible within the IDS's financial capacity, as discussed in Chapter 8. A related form of sustainability relates to the ability of the plan to promote physician recruitment and retention by being related in perception and reality to the market. The market in this case is commonly measured by national and regional compensation surveys, including those produced by the Medical Group Management Association (MGMA), the American Medical Group Association (AMGA), and others.

Defined performance expectations and requirements

Effective plans help to clarify the expectations that an IDS has for its physicians related to productivity and work levels and in other ways. This will commonly be accomplished by explicit requirements in the physician's employment contract, but also both implicitly and explicitly through the IDS compensation and financial incentive systems.

Simple and understandable

Effective compensation plans in IDS or other settings must also be simple and understandable. This is essential given that an IDS's compensation practices are an important component of the physician performance feedback and incentive system within the IDS. Plans that are so complicated that they can't be understood by the physicians who work under them, or are difficult to administer, tend to be less effective in the long term. Effective plans also tend to be clearly defined, meaning that the plan is clearly expressed and uses objective measures and an agreed-upon set of rules that apply in a largely consistent manner.

The compensation plans used in today's successful IDS tend to embody these essential principles. These principles are the direct results of the experiences of the 1990s and the compensation practices that were generally viewed to have failed because they could not be repeated or sustained on a long-term basis.

UNDERSTANDING THE CONTEXT OF COMPENSATION IN AN INTEGRATED DELIVERY SYSTEM

Compensation arrangements tend to both reflect and influence an IDS's culture. This means that changes to a compensation plan will influence an IDS's culture. Where changes to the IDS culture are desired, the change process will commonly include decisions to change the underlying physician compensation arrangements and practices.

The unique nature of the IDS environment is the involvement of organizations, such as hospitals and health systems, that are, by definition, different from those involved in a typical physician-owned "private practice" setting. In a private practice setting, the physician has a direct alignment with the organization that the physician owns, or at a minimum, has a close relationship and sense of control over the private practice entity as the "physician's practice." A true private practice setting frequently provides the framework for teamwork and a potentially greater sense of the economic reality that all of the group's providers are "in it together" in financial terms.

In an IDS, direct employment by a hospital, health system, or physician practice organization is the essential nature of the underlying relationship because the physicians are employees of the IDS. As a result, the financial and other relationships between the physician and the IDS are frequently different than in a true private practice. In an IDS, the physicians are not true owners of the system, so their bottom line compensation is not as directly linked to the IDS's overall financial performance and success.

Instead of a partnership, IDS physicians have a one-to-one or employer–employee relationship with a component of the system (for example, the hospital, captive practice entity, or other organization), and this results in compensation for an individual physician being determined by a direct one-on-one negotiation with the physician's employer. Therefore, the success or failure of other physicians within the same organization may, or may not, have any direct implications for physician compensation and performance. As a result, a common challenge in the context of IDS compensation plan development is to develop and maintain models that promote a level of both individual and group-wide accountability and financial performance that will promote the success of the organization as a whole, even though the essential nature of the relationship involves employment of individual physicians by the IDS.

Whereas in the true private practice, all physicians are "in it together" the fact that each is, at the end, an employee of a larger system, will sometimes make it more difficult to balance team and individual incentives. Promoting this accountability is commonly made more difficult by the fact that from an individual physician's perspective, the IDS will always be viewed as having greater access to financial resources and "deep pockets" to pay compensation.

BASIC PLAN TYPES

There are as many different types of IDS compensation plans as there are types of integrated systems. Nonetheless, the plan methods may be classified into a number of basic models that adopt different approaches to the determination of physician compensation. In today's environment, virtually all models involve a significant focus on production and productivity at the individual, group, or combined levels. Thus, almost all models have a significant production component, although the manner in which production is measured and related to compensation paid varies considerably.

Within productivity-based models, most compensation plans tend to involve a largely individualistic approach that treats each individual physician as a largely separate unit for compensation purposes. However, some integrated systems adopt and implement compensation practices that tend to be team-oriented through which compensation and/or financial conditions at a larger practice-wide level are considered. In these models the effort of the practice site and/or team will be measured and assessed in determining compensation. The result of that assessment will commonly impact some or all of the compensation available to the physicians working within the particular practice group.

Physician-specific or "individualistic" models

Individualistic compensation models tend to treat each individual physician as a largely separate unit for compensation plan purposes. The compensation plan measures individual physician performance to determine the individual physician's compensation for his or her services. Physician work or production may be measured through a variety of means including actual collections for professional services, percentage of gross or net charges, work relative value units (RVUs), or other means. Likewise, many (but certainly not all) IDS compensation plans using individualistic models also consider practice operating costs or overhead.

Individualistic models tend to be utilized in all types of integrated systems. They also tend to be perceived as most desirable and appropriate in those practices in which there is significant variation among physicians in terms of production, specialization, work levels, and related issues. They make each individual physician responsible and accountable for his or her own work or production level, and potentially for a share of practice overhead.

Group-oriented models

Group-oriented models tend to treat a set of related physician practices within the IDS as a single unit for purposes of some or all of the physician's compensation. A compensation pool may be developed by combining the amount of money otherwise due and payable to individual physicians under more individualistic, physician-specific compensation plans, but that pool may then be real located or redistributed among the practice group's physicians in a manner that meets their collective goals. Some team or group-oriented models calculate some "net amount" at a practice or group level by the consideration of revenues, expenses, or a combination thereof, and the plan distributes the net among a subset of the IDS's physicians. These methods often attempt to consider the practice's overall overhead expenses as a cost of doing business — the expenses are considered at a group rather than an individual physician level.

Within group-oriented models, any number of measures and combination of measures for measuring work or production — professional service charges, net or gross charges, work RVUs, and other methods — might be combined with an equal share, base salary, or similar component.

The utility of group-oriented models is that they have the potential to promote a practice group-wide perspective. Because these models encourage production and/or managing costs for the good of the practice group or team, they can help ensure that all physicians in a single practice or setting focus on "rowing together." These models tend to work well in single-specialty practices within an IDS, as well as in other practices where there are not wide variations between physicians' work levels.

THE ROLE OF PRODUCTION AND PRODUCTIVITY

A central theme in virtually all compensation plans in a successful IDS is an appropriate level of attention to productivity and work in determining and paying physician compensation. The culture of production and productivity is expressed in the compensation plan and in the organization's approach to doing business. IDS compensation plans tend to measure physician production or work through any number of means.

Four broad categories of measures of physician work or "production" are commonly used in compensation plans used in integrated systems today:

- Gross charges from professional services;
- Net revenues from professional charges (net of contractual adjustments);
- Collections from professional services, defined as the actual cash received by the practice from the activities of an individual physician; and
- RVUs involving an objective measure of work and effort defined by Medicare or other organizations.

Just as there is no perfect compensation plan, there is no completely perfect or correct metric to be used to allocate practice revenues. For example, charges represent no more than the "asking price" for services, so there is no direct relationship between cash on hand and the value of the amount charged for the services rendered. Nonetheless, many integrated systems determine compensation by basing the amount paid on a percentage of professional service charges, in large part because charges are payer neutral and well understood by IDS physicians.

Collections have the value and benefit that they relate to the actual money received by the IDS for a physician's services, but where collections are used, issues of payer mix and collection performance (by the IDS itself) will come into play.

Work or total relative value units or RVUs use a standard measure to determine and pay physician compensation. Most RVU-based compensation plans incorporate the Medicare Resource-Based Relative Value Scale (RBRVS) RVUs as the basis for determining reimbursement for physician services. The RBRVS system was developed, in part, as a means to provide uniform payment for the same services, while taking into account variations and the cost of service provision in different parts of the country. RBRVS assigns relative value units to individual Current Procedural Terminology (CPT®)* codes for Medicare payment purposes, with separate values assigned for:

- Physician work;
- Practice expenses; and
- Malpractice expenses.

Many physicians' compensation plans today use the work RVU component for purposes of determining compensation levels. Many integrated systems elect to use work RVUs, in whole or in part, in compensation plans because they measure work in a more objective manner than charges or collections. Thus, the use of work RVUs in a compensation plan may have value because it enables an organization to reward work without regard to payer mix, reimbursement levels, or other factors.

Where RVUs are used to define the relationship to physician productivity, it will be important to recognize that periodic changes in RVU values by the Centers for Medicare & Medicaid Services (CMS) are likely to result in unexpected increases or decreases in physician compensation levels. For example, many RBRVS work RVU values were changed in connection with the 2007 Medicare Physician Fee Schedule in a manner that both created considerable confusion and had significant financial implications in many settings. In that year, the two changes combined to have a significant impact on RVU values.

One change was required by provisions of the Social Security Act, which governs the Medicare program and requires a periodic review of the work RVUs and the methodology for calculating practice expenses within the RBRVS system. These changes resulted in substantial increases in the RVU values assigned to evaluation and management (E&M) services and certain other services. For example, the work RVU values associated with CPT code 99213 (intermediate outpatient office visit) increased from 0.67 RVUs in the 2006 Medicare Physician Fee Schedule to 0.92 RVUs in the 2007 Fee Schedule, constituting a 37 percent increase in the work credit for the procedure, without any change to the aggregate reimbursement provided by Medicare (through the combination of the work, practice expense, and malpractice components that are combined to determine total RVUs and used to determine reimbursement from the Medicare program).

The second change that occurred in 2007 was the imposition of a statutorily mandated "budget neutrality factor" under the Medicare program. This factor is designed to ensure that the amount of reimbursement provided by the U.S. government for Medicare services stays within certain budgetary parameters. In 2007, the budget neutrality factor combined with the increase in work RVU values for E&M and certain other codes resulted in a *reduction* in reimbursement for all work RVU reimbursement rates by approximately 10 percent. Put otherwise, the work credit assigned to certain RVUs increased but without any actual increase in the reimbursement paid for that work.

As a result of these changes, where work RVUs are used to determine and pay physician compensation, certain physicians (especially primary care) may commonly benefit in the form of increased work credit (measured by work RVUs) in the compensation plan. This is illustrated in market survey data for primary care specialties such that is found in the MGMA's *Physician Compensation and Production Survey: 2006 Report Based on 2005 Data*[1] summarized in Exhibit 7.1. Exhibit 7.1 illustrates the dramatic changes for family practice physicians that occurred with the release of the 2007 Medicare Physician Fee Schedule. For family practice physicians (without obstetrics), the median number of encounters, collections from professional services, and compensation remained largely

EXHIBIT 7.1 ■ Effect of Medicare Physician Fee Schedule Changes on Family Physicians (Without Obstetrics), 2006–2007

	Family Practice (Without Obstetrics)			
Description	**2006**	**Reporting Physicians**	**2007**	**Reporting Physicians**
Work RVU Units	4,073[1]	2,365	4,600[2]	3,629
$ Value/Work Unit	$41.04	2,339	$38.89[2]	3,629
Encounters	4,051	4,215	4,055	4,206
Compensation	$164,021	5,850	$173,812[2]	5,959
Collections (profit)	$367,744	2,597	$363,214	2,463

RVU — relative value unit
[1] *Federal Register*, vol. 70, no. 223 (November 21, 2005).
[2] *Federal Register*, vol. 72, no. 236 (December 10, 2006).

constant, but the number of work RVUs increased significantly for the physicians reporting to the survey.

Where an IDS or another medical practice pays a pre-assigned dollar amount per work RVU under the physician pay formula (such as $41.04 per RVU using data from Exhibit 7.1) without making any adjustment for the change in work RVU value credit (or reimbursement received under Medicare reimbursement), the physicians paid under such arrangement would receive a significant financial windfall — even though the IDS (or medical practice) received no more reimbursement for the physician's work. For example, using data from Exhibit 7.1, a physician who produced 4,073 work RVUs and was paid $41.04 (using 2006 data) would receive total compensation of $167,155. However, if the same dollar amount of $41.04 per RVU was used in 2007, the increased number of work RVUs at the median level (4,600) would yield total compensation of $188,784 for the same level of work.

Despite these points, work RVUs are not inherently problematic, and in fact, many IDS compensation plans use work RVUs to measure work and physician production because they are payer neutral and objective. Yet these changes and this illustration demonstrate the importance of considering changes in the values in connection with IDS physician compensation plans. This highlights the need to incorporate provisions in any formula that will permit flexibility to avoid major fluctuations that could prove to be financially adverse to either the physician or the IDS.

THE ROLE OF PRACTICE OPERATING COSTS

Some but not all IDS compensation practices involve some form of direct cost of practice consideration at the individual physician or group level. Of course, because compensation practices within an IDS must be sustainable, cost of practice will always need to be considered in some manner within the IDS. Where the costs are considered indirectly, they are assessed at a high level by the organization in evaluating whether the compensation practices are affordable and sustainable in light of the system's revenue base, compensation and benefit costs, and other practice-related overhead.

Where costs are considered explicitly, IDS compensation plans will commonly take different approaches to such an explicit cost allocation. Some models allocate costs based upon an agreed-upon "cost accounting" or similar methods. In these plans, costs within a practice are tracked and allocated among practice physicians. For example, some integrated systems divide costs into categories of:

- Fixed costs (those that are generally fixed in nature for such things as facilities and equipment);
- Variable costs (costs that vary based upon resource utilization or production); and
- Direct expense items that are typically consumed by, and allocated directly to, individual physicians.

Variable expense items are often allocated on a fully variable or a combined fixed variable cost basis. Thus, personnel costs, supplies, and the like may have a portion allocated equally among all physicians and the remaining portion allocated based upon a percentage of production — physicians who have higher production will bear a larger share of the expense.

Direct expenses include items such as professional liability insurance costs, continuing medical education expenses, and physician-specific business expenses. These direct costs are allocated directly to individual physicians as part of the compensation calculation.

Some systems also allocate the physician's "personal" support personnel such as a medical assistant, a physician assistant, or other provider. Because the physician will most commonly receive the credit for the extender's work and performance, the physician will also commonly bear the associated risk and expense.

Quality, satisfaction, and other measures

In addition to the basic financial model involving some allocation of revenues and expenses discussed earlier, many integrated systems use other, more intangible or subjective measures to allocate at least a portion of physician compensation. These systems often focus on issues of patient satisfaction, quality, financial, or other performance at a subgroup level, such as a department or practice site. Compensation committees, quality review boards, objective patient satisfaction scores in relation to targeted levels of performance, and similar measures are used to allocate a defined pool of money available for compensation. Often these measures are also used to reward money that has already been earmarked for individual performance.

Likewise, measures focusing on group-level financial or other performance typically provide for the allocation of defined dollar amounts (commonly based upon a percentage of base salary or the like) for performance in relation to defined targets or goals. The targets and goals often include financial performance as well as performance related to practice growth and outreach, patient access standards, and increased patient visit volumes. In most instances, performance is evaluated by reference to agreed-upon criteria, with an award of a defined level of compensation that is based on performance in relation to a target.

IDS COMPENSATION PLAN EXAMPLES

As stated earlier in this chapter, there is no perfect compensation plan, only alternative compensation plans that are more or less perfect for an IDS and its group of physicians at a particular point in time. The challenge in crafting the appropriate compensation plan for a particular IDS is to craft a plan that reasonably promotes the system's goals (for example, sustainability, recruitment, and retention), while also maintaining a reasonable level of physician satisfaction. The basic methodological tools outlined in the previous sections can be thought of as building blocks to use in crafting the arrangement that will work for the IDS at a particular point in time.

This section reviews and illustrates many of the compensation systems used in integrated systems today. Multiple examples are provided, and in each instance the individual plan is likely to involve both the technical plan methodology referenced as follows, along with additional details to show precisely how the plan would work in an IDS. Keep in mind that different aspects of the plans illustrated here can be mixed and matched in different compensation arrangements. This means, for example, that a base salary plus production-based incentive system illustrated in one example could be combined with other incentive measures focusing on cost, quality, patient satisfaction, or other objectives. Likewise, many of the various "technical details" described as follows could also be combined with the basic methodologies outlined here.

Base-plus-incentive compensation plans

Many IDSs use "base-plus-incentive" or "XYZ" compensation systems, in which the base salary is determined through the use of various factors, including by linking the actual payment to market levels of compensation for the practice specialty, the individual physician's historic compensation levels, or determined in some other manner. The base amount often varies by the physician's specialty, years of practice, production, or other factors. The base salary frequently comprises only a subset of the estimated total compensation, with the additional or "incentive" component determined and paid based upon other factors. Market data such as surveys from the MGMA, AMGA, and other sources are often used to establish base salary levels related to physician specialties, work levels, and/or other factors. Also, the base salary may typically be linked to market data for particular physician practice specialty and coupled with clearly defined performance expectations regarding work levels, citizenship, and other factors.

Often incentive compensation is added on top of the base salary guarantee and measured through the use of work RVUs, gross charges, or collections from professional services. Exhibit 7.2 provides an example of a base-salary-plus-incentive model with production-based incentive compensation paid for work

RVU production in excess of a target. The incentive compensation amount may also be linked to market data. An example is those methods that pay median dollars per work RVU for production in excess of median production levels for the practice specialty.

As shown in Exhibit 7.2, these methods often involve pre-established targets to permit the system to pay additional production-based compensation for work that exceeds the predefined target. Additional incentive measures are also sometimes added on top of the production-based measures for performance in relation to quality, patient satisfaction, and other factors.

Exhibit 7.3 also illustrates a base-salary-plus-incentive model, but it uses gross production from professional services for purposes of incentive compensation in that it awards a predefined percentage of gross professional charges in relation to target amounts. Exhibit 7.3 also illustrates the application of additional incentive measures including the potential award of additional compensation based on quality, patient satisfaction, or other measures.

EXHIBIT 7.2 ■ Base Salary Plus Incentive, Example 1

Base and Incentive

▪ Base set at MGMA survey median for specialty.	Base	$ 150,000
▪ Must meet MGMA median wRVU production. If missed, Base Salary is unchanged.	$ per RVU	$ 41.50
▪ RVU Target calculated by dividing Base Salary by MGMA median work RVU conversion factor.	RVU Target	3,614
▪ Incentive conversion per work RVU paid at MGMA 50th percentile conversion factor for specialty.	50th percentile	$ 47.50
▪ Production over target paid at 50th percentile conversion factor.		
Example		
▪ Base Salary = $150,000	Base	$ 150,000
▪ Target = 3,614 work RVU		
▪ $ per work RVU Over Target = $47.50	RVU Target	3,614
▪ Actual work RVU Production = 3,849	Actual RVUs	3,849
▪ Difference From Target = 235	RVUs Above Target	235
	$ Per RVU	$ 47.50
	Incentive	$ 11,163
	Total Compensation	$ 161,163

MGMA — Medical Group Management Association
RVU — relative value unit

EXHIBIT 7.3 ■ Base Salary Plus Incentive, Example 2

Methodology

- Base salary defined in agreement
- Performance requirements for direct GPC no less than $528,000
- Target for GPC equal to $423,000
- Productivity incentive (physician is paid a defined percentage of GPC in excess of target using tiers above GPC Target):
  - First $47,999 over target = 31.1%
  - $48,000–98,999 over target = 33.2%
  - $99,000–150,999 over target = 39.0%
  - $151,000–209,999 over target = 41.8%
  - Over $210,000 and target = 46.1%
- Practice bonus principles (eligible to receive Principles of Practice Bonus up to $10,000 in four categories):
  - Cost control (30%)
  - Leadership/collaboration (10%)
  - Customer satisfaction (40%)
  - Clinical focus (20%)
- Beat-budget incentive compensation (if the practice breaks even, the physician is eligible for an end-of-year Beat-Budget Bonus)

Example

- Base salary = $110,000
- GPC = $580,000
- Receives increasing portions in excess of GPC target

Dr. A			
GPC	$580,000		
Base salary	$ 110,000		
Incentive compensation			
GPC target	$423,000		
$ 47,999		31.10%	$ 14,928
$ 98,999		33.20%	$ 16,932
$ 99,000		39.00%	$ 20,280
$ 151,000		41.80%	$ 2,508
$ 210,000		46.10%	
Total Compensation Dr. A			$164,647

GPC — gross professional charges

Exhibit 7.4 also illustrates a base-salary-plus-incentive model. In Exhibit 7.4, compensation is determined on a quarterly basis throughout the year. This example therefore involves a guaranteed base salary coupled with quarterly evaluations in relation to physician production during the quarter. Production is measured through the use of total RVUs in relation to a target (with the target determined in relation to the base salary). Where the physician has production in excess of the target, the incentive is earned. Exhibit 7.4 also illustrates a blending of different market survey values for a particular practice specialty to determine the dollar amount per total RVU paid under the model.

Practice operating costs can also be considered in some manner in connection with base-plus-incentive compensation models as shown in Exhibit 7.5.

EXHIBIT 7.4 ■ Guaranteed Base Plus Incentive

Base and Incentive Compensation	*Example*	
▪ Base salary set at defined level (e.g., $400,000)	Mean	$ 24.40
▪ Incentive paid where $ per Total RVU (TRVU) x TRVU production exceeds base salary	25th	$ 21.34
	Median	$ 25.45
▪ Incentive compensation comp/TRVU conversion factor calculated at average of 25th percentile, Mean, Median, 75th percentile, and 90th percentile using MGMA survey data for specialty	75th	$ 26.98
	90th	$ 28.29
	Average	$ 25.29
Example		
▪ TRVU for quarter	TRVU	3,450.00
▪ TRVU x conversion factor = compensation earned	$ per TRVU	$ 25.29
▪ Base salary = $400,000 ($100,000 per quarter)	Total for quarter	$ 87,250
▪ Physician compensation using $ per TRVU does not meet base compensation for quarter, so he/she receives base only ($100,000)		

RVU — relative value unit
TRVU — total RVUs

In this model, the base salary is set based on practice-wide financial performance. Incentive is paid in the form of a predefined portion of any overage of practice revenues in excess of allocated expenses. This model requires the physician to effectively cover his or her direct base-salary compensation and benefit costs and the allocated share of practice overhead before any incentive will be paid. Importantly, in a tax-exempt setting, this type of model requires close attention in light of concerns about tax-exempt status.

EXHIBIT 7.5 ■ Base Plus Incentive with Expense Consideration

Base Salary	*Example*	
▪ Set in relation to NPR in prior period	Under $350,000	= $120,000
▪ NPR includes revenues from direct professional services (including managed care bonus/ deficit), excluding ancillary services	$350,001–$400,000	= $140,000
	Over $401,000	= $160,000

Incentive Compensation
- Equal to NPR less allocated practice-related expenses
- If net surplus, the physician receives
  - 15% of first $15,000
  - 75% of next up to $50,000
  - 80% of remainder over $50,000

NPR — net practice revenues

Base salary plus tiered production

A variation on the previous examples involves a base salary coupled with a tiered, or graduated, incentive payment based on production. The incentive may be measured through the use of work RVUs or total RVUs that are personally performed by the physician. Such models combine the base salary component (which is commonly guaranteed) with a tiered payment for production in excess of a predefined target. The predefined targets are frequently linked to market data, thereby permitting payment for production above predefined levels. The setting of the target and conversion factor is often linked so that the combination of the guaranteed base payment and the production-based incentive compensation will yield median, similar, or other predefined levels of compensation in relation to work. Thus, median work will typically yield median compensation. This type of approach to compensation is illustrated in Exhibit 7.6, which combines a base salary for primary care physicians with a graduated dollar amount per work RVU for production in excess of defined targets.

In many IDS's pay formulas, instead of linking the dollar amount per work RVU to reported MGMA, AMGA, or similar values, the compensation system uses a calculation approach to determine a starting point "conversion factor"

EXHIBIT 7.6 ■ Tiered Work RVU Production, Primary Care Model

Primary Care Model

- Specialty-specific
- Base compensation guaranteed
- Three tiers
- Three conversion factor tiers
- FTE status
- $ per work RVU paid based on production per year

Example

- Full-time Internal Medicine
- Full-time equivalent
- Actual RVUs = 5,547

	RVU	$ per RVU	Dr. A
Actual RVUs			5,547
Base compensation			$90,000.00
Tier 1	3,812	$ 47.50	$18,430.00
Tier 1	4,200	$ 51.60	$15,480.00
Tier 1	4,500	$ 58.40	$61,144.80
Total compensation			$185,054.80

Pass Through Items

- Performance payments
- Mid-level supervision payments
- "Outside income"

RVU — relative value unit

for physician compensation. In essence, the common theme is that median work levels should yield median compensation. Thus, median compensation levels as measured by the market will be divided by median work RVUs to determine the calculated level of compensation per work RVU at the median level of production.

Such methodologies reward physicians for their work without regard to payment levels, payer mix, or related factors. Likewise, the linkage to market data provides a level of internal and external validity to the dollar amount paid per work RVU. As with any system, however, the primary challenge is to set the dollar-per-work RVU conversion factor at a level that is acceptable, while also ensuring that the organization has sufficient revenues to fund the compensation.

Direct linkage to market data

Some integrated systems directly link physician production levels to reported market data values as set forth in MGMA, AMGA, or other market surveys. The theory is that productivity at the 25th percentile will result in compensation equal to the reported 25th percentile values, and so on. Thus, the compensation plan will be directly linked to the survey in a lockstep fashion.

While commonly used, such a methodology frequently presents inherent challenges on two primary fronts. First, because compensation and production data in the MGMA and other survey reports do not directly correlate, a direct linkage of median compensation to median reported compensation per unit of work often results in physician compensation that is in excess of reported values. By illustration, if the median compensation value reported in MGMA data is $150,000, this does not mean that the product of the reported dollar amount per work RVU at the median level multiplied by the median number of work RVUs will yield $150,000. In fact, the product of such measures often yields a number that exceeds the reported median value. As a result of this reality of market data, integrated systems often pay more than they expect where direct linkage to market data occurs. Instead of such direct linkage, many integrated systems elect to calculate the dollar amount per work value by dividing reported compensation values by reported production values to derive their own calculated conversion factor.

The second inherent challenge of using a compensation formula directly linked to market data is that the data, by nature, are imprecise and inexact. As the product of self-report surveys, market data are subject to variation from year to year and, depending on the table or cut of data used, will even vary within the same published survey report (for example, the "all physician" values will differ from those for the particular region, hospital affiliated practices, and so on). This variation often creates challenges for the IDS and the physicians who are looking for some level of stability of income and cash flow from year to year. As a result, many integrated systems will use an average of multiple values (averaging median values from several survey tables in MGMA, AMGA, and other reports) to provide for some level of year-to-year stability so as to prevent wide fluctuations based upon year-to-year changes in market data and inconsistencies in the survey's data.

This type of direct linkage is illustrated in Exhibit 7.7, which uses different RVU payment rates based on production in relation to MGMA data. While feasible, this type of model may have challenges due to the changes in market data and due to the absence of a direct relationship between compensation and production percentiles in market survey information. On the other hand, such models can be useful in the near term to stimulate greater attention to, and incremental improvement in, work and production levels, in particular where the IDS physicians tend to have below-median production levels. Exhibit 7.7 also illustrates other potential adjustments to compensation, including adjustments for electronic medical record implementation (short term), compensation for leadership, and treatment of income from outside activities.

EXHIBIT 7.7 ■ Direct Link to MGMA Data

Production Compensation

- Compensation per work RVU linked directly to MGMA percentiles by specialty

Example

25th percentile = 34.55
30th percentile = 35.66
35th percentile = 36.69
40th percentile = 37.53
45th percentile = 38.08
50th percentile = 38.89
55th percentile = 39.90
60th percentile = 40.99
65th percentile = 44.30
70th percentile = 44.03
75th percentile = 45.95

EMR Implementation Adjustment

- 100% production first 60 days
- 90% production next 30 days
- Requirements regarding days worked, etc.

Facilities Compensation

- Contract income from nursing home, correctional facility, etc.
- Taxed at inverse of cost of taxes, Social Security and other withholdings, and benefit costs (for example, 75.46%)
- No work RVU credit

Leadership Compensation

- No work RVU credit
- Stipend per month

EMR — electronic medical record
MGMA — Medical Group Manangment Association
RVU — relative value unit

Pure production with tiered payment levels

Many compensation systems involve pure production-based approaches, but they couple this with differential payment levels for production in excess of defined targets. Such systems frequently use tiers or graduated payments per work RVU, percentages of gross charges, or other factors. These tiers are a means to recognize that given the operating costs in a practice, low levels of production typically yield lower amounts that can be paid in the form of compensation while high levels of production typically yield greater compensation due to the fact that much of the practice operating costs have been covered.

Exhibits 7.8 and 7.9 illustrate two approaches to the setting of tiers and the assignment of payment levels to each tier. Exhibit 7.8 illustrates a pure production model that uses an historic rolling 12-month average to determine the level of RVU payment for physician work during a defined period. The tiers and grid in this example are calculated using median compensation and work RVU data from market survey (with median compensation divided by median RVUs to determine the "median" or 100 percent value in the grid). Values that are from 80 to 120 percent of this composite median value are then calculated and used to award different compensation levels for different production in relation to market levels.

EXHIBIT 7.8 ■ Pure Production RVU Grid Model

Production-Based Compensation

- Comp/work RVU based on grid/matrix of work RVU values (e.g., 80% of median, 85% of median, 90% of median, 95% of median, 105% of median, 110% of median, 115% of median, 120% of median)
- Physician paid defined compensation per RVU based on production level (e.g., using rolling average for 12 months or other period)

Example

% of Median	$ per work RVU
80%	$ 33.20
85%	$ 35.28
90%	$ 37.35
95%	$ 39.43
100%	$ 41.50
105%	$ 43.58
110%	$ 45.65
115%	$ 47.73
120%	$ 49.80

Example

- Rolling 12-month average work RVU production equal to 97% of median for subject pay period (e.g., 1-month period)
- Dr. A produces 547 work RVUs during pay period
- Dr. A is paid $39.43 per work RVU during pay period (equal to 95% of median on grid/matrix of work RVU values)

Work RVUs	547
$ per work RVU	$ 39.43
Period compensation	$ 21,568

RVU — relative value unit

EXHIBIT 7.9 ■ Tiered Work RVU Production

	Example
Dollar per Work RVU ▪ Dollars per work RVU paid based on production per year ▪ Five tiers	Annual work RVUs Under 80% of benchmark = $45 80% to 3,900 = $52 3,901 to 4,700 = $55 4,401 to 5,700 = $57 Over 5,700 = 65
Quality Measures ▪ Additional compensation for performance in relation to three quality measures: diabetes, coronary artery disease, and heart failure ▪ Three benchmarks per individual quality measure, all of which must be met to be compensated for the quality measure ▪ Total available is linked to work RVU production and number of benchmarks met:	Total available per quarter based on work RVUs (subject to additional adjustment for number of quality measures met)
— 1 quality measure met = 20% of total based on work RVUs — 2 quality measures met = 50% of total based on work RVUs — 3 quality measures met = 100% of total based on work RVUs	Under 975 work RVUs = $1,250 976 to 1,175 work RVUs = $1,875 1,176 to 1,425 work RVUs = $2,500 Over 1,425 work RVUs = $3,750
Timing ▪ Compensation reviewed once per year ▪ Base is set at 90% of estimated compensation based on production ▪ Physician repayment for "overpayments"	

RVU — relative value unit

Exhibit 7.9 also illustrates a tiered dollars-per-RVU model, but it involves fewer tiers or steps. It also illustrates the consideration of quality factors, but links the payment rates to production levels.

Compensation systems that use tiered RVU or other values recognize implicitly that there is a correlation between work levels and overhead rates, or operating costs, associated with a particular practice. A physician whose production would place him or her at the 25th percentile, as measured by MGMA or other market data, would produce lower levels of revenues and would typically have a higher overhead rate (expressed as a percentage of total revenues produced) than a colleague producing at the 50th or 75th percentiles. Because the largest portion of medical practice costs are fixed, the lower-producing physician will need to cover his or her costs before receiving additional amounts in the form of compensation. Thus, under these RVU methodologies, a graduated scale is typically used to pay increasing dollar amounts per work RVU that are themselves linked to physician production.

Tiered percentage of professional charges

A variation of the pure production-based approach to compensation uses gross charges from professional services on a direct percentage of production or tiered percentage basis to determine physician pay levels. In such models, the IDS standard charge schedule for professional services is used as the starting point, and physicians are paid a predefined percentage of their personally performed professional service charges in the form of compensation (for example, 30 percent of all professional service charges, or a "tiered" amount, such as 25 percent of the first $200,000 of professional service charges, 30 percent of $200,000 to $400,000 of professional service charges, and 35 percent of all professional service charges in excess of $400,000).

As with all other models, the particular percentages and approach must be tailored to consider practice specialty and services. Thresholds for general surgeons will therefore vary significantly from those established for primary care or other specialties. Such models also must consider physician cash flow and will therefore commonly include the production-based model with a base salary or a salary advance or draw to provide for stability of payments throughout the year. Such payments are periodically (quarterly, every six months, and annually) reconciled to ensure that physician compensation aligns with actual production and compensation earned under the pay plan.

This type of approach is illustrated in Exhibit 7.10, in which the bulk of compensation is based on professional service production. Note that due to its approach to the consideration and distribution of ancillary services, Exhibit 7.10 would be feasible only in an IDS that uses a true group practice legal structure. Thus, this model would only be available in a captive or separate group practice legal entity within the IDS; it wound not be available for use in direct employment relationships with hospitals or health systems. Exhibit 7.10 also illustrates other potential tools in compensation systems, including system-wide bonuses and similar measures.

Cost-of-practice models

In compensation systems that consider practice operating expenses, the IDS focuses both on incentivising and rewarding production, while also mirroring private practice by promoting greater physician responsibility and accountability for practice expenses. One common approach is to attribute revenue production to professional services performed by the individual physician. An attributed net revenue is therefore determined by multiplying the professional service charges by a predefined percentage (for example, 50 percent or 65 percent depending upon the specialty). This attributed net revenue amount may or may not correspond directly with the actual collections from the physician's professional service performance. Such an approach has the benefit of being payer neutral such that physicians receive the same level of revenue credit regardless of payer mix.

EXHIBIT 7.10 ■ Tiered Percent of Professional Collections with Expense Consideration

	Example		
Tiered Percent of Professional Collections ▪ Graduated scale of payment to physician as percent of professional service collections (excluding ancillary and midlevel provider supervision) — 1st $200,000 = 45% to physician — $200,001 to 260,000 = 55% — Over $260,001 = 70% ▪ Adjusted net collections percentage guaranteed to be no less than 90% and no greater than 110%. If actual is outside of this range, then closest value is used (e.g., if actual = 89%, then 90% would be used to calculate professional collections) ▪ Financial management system tracks professional collections, non-professional collections (including ancillaries), and expenses (with expenses designed to mirror those in private practice)	Actual professional collections		$324,405
	1st $200,000	45%	$ 90,000
	$200,001 to 260,000	55%	$ 33,000
	Over $260,001	70%	$ 45,084
			$168,084
Ancillary Service Income ▪ Ancillary service pools for each clinic ▪ Pool funded at 50% of non-professional collections (ancillary service collections) from clinic ▪ Each physician allocated a percentage of pool based on percent of professional service collections	Non-professional collections (clinic)		$ 105,094
	Pool (clinic)		$ 52,547
	% of total		23%
	Non-professional collections share		$ 12,125
Midlevel Supervision ▪ 8% of total professional and non-professional collections	Midlevel collections		$ 128,982
	8% of collections		8.00%
	Midlevel supervision pay		$ 10,319
Practice Profit (Loss) ▪ Primary care physicians have predefined level of system subsidy (loss) per year: — Years 1 to 3 = $65,000 — Year 4 = $50,000 — Year 5 and after = $30,000 ▪ Total net income from practice equals (professional collections + non-professional collections) – expenses ▪ Profit (loss) compared to predefined level of system support per year: — If loss is less than predefined level, physician receives difference — If loss is greater than predefined level, loss allocated to physician	System support max		$ 30,000
	Profit (loss)		$ 28,983
	Difference		$ 1,017
Total Compensation ▪ Sum of amounts above	Tiered % of professional collections		$168,084
	Ancillary		$ 12,125
	Midlevel supervision		$ 10,319
	System profit (loss)		$ 1,017
	Total compensation		$191,544

On top of the attributed net revenues some attribution of practice operating expenses will also be considered. Operating expenses are often categorized into what are frequently referred to as *controllable operating expenses* for staff, space and equipment, and related costs. Such controllable operating expenses are commonly categorized as fixed, variable, and direct expenses (consideration will be given to the extent to which the actual expenses that are allocated are consistent with those that would be expected in a private practice setting). Adjustments to the expense allocation formula will therefore be made for special circumstances such as the placement of physicians in hospital-quality office space, even though a private practice model is in place with lower operating costs. Likewise, some consideration of the typically more expensive hospital employee benefit structure will also frequently occur in defining attributed operating costs.

The compensation plan in such instances typically involves a revenues-minus-expense calculation method, with the physician earning compensation based upon the difference between the two. Such a model has inherent value in that it mimics private practice to a greater extent than other models by considering actual or attributed operating expenses. Because of the model's consideration of actual or attributed net revenues, however, close attention to legal compliance is essential where the IDS is operated as a tax exempt, Section 501(c)(3) organization. (An example of this type of model is shown in Exhibit 7.11.)

"Group" or "practice site" specific net revenue: Expense model

An additional variation on the revenues-minus-expense model referenced in the previous section measures performance at a "group" or "practice site" level. This model also typically involves an attribution or actual tracking of net revenues or actual collections from professional and other services. Ancillary services and the performance of non-physician providers may only be considered in models used in a true group practice setting such as those involving a captive subsidiary group practice entity within the IDS. This is because the Stark Law's in-office ancillary services exception, while permitting the tracking and crediting of non-physician performance including ancillary services, is only available for use in a true group practice setting.

In these models, revenues and expenses associated with the practice are tracked at an individual and at a group level. A practice (such as the family practice division or an individual practice site within a larger group practice entity) will be treated as a group, with the pay plan effectively involving the distribution of funds remaining after practice-specific expenses have been subtracted from practice net revenues. Such models are the closest to true "private practice models." While feasible, such models must be scrutinized closely in light of applicable legal requirements under the Stark Law, rules for tax-exempt organizations, and other requirements. As a result, these models arguably involve higher levels of complexity and compliance risk.

Exhibit 7.11 provides an example of such a model. Importantly, this model is used in a true "group practice" setting that consists of a single legal entity that is capable of furnishing and billing for ancillary health care services.

EXHIBIT 7.11 ■ Practice Site Professional Collections with Expense Consideration

Methodology

- Practice site professional collections
- Practice site ancillary collections
- Subsidy/variances
- Total cash collections
- Staff
- Staff and physician benefits
- Malpractice
- Rent
- Information-related expenses
- Other operating expenses (collections – operating expenses = operating expense before physician compensation)

  Divided among physicians at site based upon (option):
  - Professional charges
  - Work RVUs

Thresholds can be used to reflect economics of private practice and disproportionately reward higher production

Example

- Designed to reward higher production
- Different thresholds of professional production credit at different levels to provide higher weight or credit to higher levels of professional service production
  - First $200,000 = 25% weight
  - $200,001 to $300,000 = 50%
  - $300,001 to $400,000 = 75%
  - Over $400,001 = 100%

	Example Weight	Dr. A	Dr. B
Professional charges		$600,000	$350,000
First $200,000	25%	$ 50,000	$ 50,000
$200,001 to $300,000	50%	$ 50,000	$ 50,000
$300,001 to $400,000	75%	$ 75,000	$ 37,500
Over $400,001	100%	$200,000	$
Weighted credit		$375,000	$137,500
% of operating margin		73%	27%
Total operating margin	$325,000	$237,805	$ 87,195

RVU — relative value unit

In Exhibit 7.11, the total amount available for compensation is determined at the group level based on a consideration of group revenues and expenses. The compensation model effectively distributes the funds available after this calculation through an agreed upon means, with significant consideration of individual physician production levels.

ADDITIONAL TECHNICAL DETAILS

In addition to the basic plan architectures and examples referenced earlier in this chapter, IDS physician compensation plans must address a series of important technical details, including many of the issues and approaches described here.

Physician cash flow

In production-based systems, physicians require appropriate advances on compensation earned to provide adequate personal cash flow. Few individuals will be able to experience wide fluctuations in take home paychecks on a bi-weekly or monthly basis. Common approaches to addressing cash flow typically involve either the use of a guaranteed level of compensation or the establishment of a salary advance or "draw" on anticipated total compensation. Either amount is often set at a predefined percentage of market rates and current or prior year earnings (typically in the range of 60 to 90 percent of such amounts, with the precise percentage determined within the IDS).

An important difference between these two methodologies of addressing cash flow relates to whether the amounts paid are guaranteed without recourse in the event that production doesn't support the payment, or whether the amount paid is subject to ultimate adjustment or reconciliation over time. Where plans have a heavy emphasis on production and productivity, the amount paid is merely a draw on amounts earned, in which case reconciliation or adjustments will be in order if the amount earned fails to meet the amount earned under the production-based compensation system.

Outside income

The bulk of any physician's time commitment is typically for the IDS, but physicians often have outside income opportunities including those involving medical directorships and research activities. In most instances, integrated systems require the full-time commitment of the physician to the organization's activities. With that commitment comes the organization's right to receive payments from all services including those performed for the organization and those outside activities that involve the practice of medicine.

Some integrated systems permit outside income to flow directly to the physician, typically with some reduction for administrative costs (for example, 10 to 15 percent). This is particularly the case when the physician performs the service during regular business hours as opposed to during weekends, evenings, vacation, or other scheduled days off. Even when the income flows to the individual physician directly, most integrated systems require disclosure of the activities, and many also require affirmative consent by the IDS for outside activities involving the practice of medicine. This disclosure is important to enable a reasonable level of monitoring of physician activities, to identify and address circumstances where the activities may be inconsistent with the IDS's values or expectations, and to minimize potential liability exposure. Another important issue in the compensation and employment relationship is whether the IDS's professional liability insurance provides coverage for outside activities. Such issues are usually addressed in the physician's employment contract.

Administrative service

Consistent with the theme of promoting physician leadership, influence, and accountability for his or her practice, many integrated systems vest significant authority in one or more physicians for administrative and practice-related activities. Such administrative service, whether in the form of a practice operations committee, an advisory body, or formal governing board, often requires the commitment of additional time and energy by the physician. Not all integrated systems pay for such administrative service. Some define it as part of the physician's regular duties and job-related requirements. When a more significant time commitment and focus is required, administrative activities may be addressed through the payment of an additional administrative stipend, typically measured and paid on an hourly basis for services actually performed. This permits the removal of the separate payment in the event that the physician ceases providing the services.

Part-time arrangements

A variety of physicians seek reduced or part-time service arrangements, such as younger physicians with children at home, mid-career physicians, and senior physicians seeking to slow down but not completely retire from their practices. The approaches to addressing part-time practice are as numerous as there are integrated systems. Some practices facilitate true "job share arrangements" in which two physicians share one full-time position including the sharing of office space, support staff, and other components of overhead. Given that physicians may work anywhere from four to five days per week, the effective use of true job share arrangements can some times yield increased productivity and resource utilization as the sum of two half-time physicians can sometimes exceed the productivity of one full-time physician.

Importantly, because part-time physicians are often still entitled to IDS benefits (health, disability, life, malpractice insurance, and other expenses), the total compensation and benefit costs of a part-time physician employee may often constitute a larger portion of the funds brought into the part-time physician's practice than in the case of full-time employees. This is generally because while the part-time physician will typically have lower levels of production, his or her benefit and practice overhead or operating costs are not always as scalable to his or her time commitment. This additional cost is sometimes included in and considered by the compensation arrangement by directly allocating the increased benefit costs to the part-time physician, thereby reducing the compensation otherwise earned.

Employee benefits

Integrated systems address employee benefit costs for health, malpractice, life, and other insurance that is advantageous to the individual physician in a variety of ways. Most integrated systems include physician benefits as a cost of doing business that is not directly allocated or attributed to the physicians themselves. The benefit costs represent a significant additional benefit to individual physicians who have previously practiced in private (physician-owned) practice settings. The IDS's provision of employee benefits therefore represents an additional level of compensation above and beyond the cash compensation provided pursuant to the compensation plan.

On the other extreme are systems that directly allocate or attribute some or all of the benefit costs to the individual physicians. Such an approach is more consistent with a "private practice" model and promotes greater physician responsibility and choice relative to the benefit structure.

TIME OFF AND PAID TIME OFF

Increasingly, integrated systems define, as part of the employment relationship, standards and expectations regarding time off for vacation, sick leave, and continuing medical education and related activities. Most integrated systems define a range of days in which the physician can be away from the practice, in part to help ensure appropriate management of practice operating expenses and overhead.

Integrated systems vary significantly in terms of their approach to separate payment for time away from the practice that is not otherwise taken. In compensation plans that use a full or largely full productivity-based system, physicians who elect to work and not take their full amount of time off will receive additional compensation through their productivity. In those systems in which a guaranteed base salary or similar guaranteed component is provided, separate payment is made for time off that is not taken (typically referred to as paid time off [PTO]), which sometimes results in payments that are above and beyond the guaranteed compensation.

While many integrated systems continue to use PTO approaches similar to those used with hospital nursing and other staff, such approaches have obvious financial implications. As a result, consistent with the increased emphasis on "private practice" compensation models in an integrated setting, integrated systems are increasingly eliminating PTO as a separate payment mechanism in most settings. The precise approach to this frequently controversial issue will often vary depending on the organization, its size, culture, and history.

Mid-level provider supervision

Dependent upon the legal and organizational structure used for the physician practice component of an IDS, mid-level provider supervision and productivity may or may not be able to be included in considering physician compensation. In particular, where the employment exception to the Stark Law is relied upon, productivity may only include the personal productivity of the employed physician. Conversely, where the IDS is able to use the Stark Law's in-office ancillary services or "group practice" exception, productivity that involves incident-to services including the services of non-physician or mid-level providers may be appropriately attributed to individual physicians or subgroups of physicians for purposes of determining physician compensation.

Increasingly, the use of the group practice type model is the exception, rather than the rule, in an IDS context. As a result, the IDS must still create incentives for physicians to provide necessary supervision and direction of mid-level providers. This is often done through an administrative or non-physician provider stipend that is linked to the number (or full-time equivalent [FTE]) of mid-level providers actually supervised. The amount of such payments will vary but may range from $5,000 to $15,000 per mid-level FTE, per year. Such payments are also typically coupled with clearly defined expectations regarding supervision, including mandatory meetings, chart review, and other activities.

Promoting quality, patient satisfaction, and related objectives

While productivity is often the primary emphasis of virtually all successful physician compensation plans, attention to other measures including quality and patient and referring physician satisfaction are also important. And while measurement of such issues is always a challenge, integrated systems increasingly devote a small portion of additional compensation that may be earned for the achievement of pre-established targets and goals related to such issues.

Quality, patient satisfaction, and other incentive measures are often funded at a predefined percentage of base or prior year pay (for example, up to 10 percent of individual physician base salary amounts). Given the objective nature of such measures, linkage to objective data, to the extent possible, is always recommended. As a result, linkage to core measures, or industry standards in a particular subspecialty (such as infection rates), is common. In all instances, the amount of money "in play" or at risk is frequently limited, but the compensation structure often permits an expansion to additional measures and additional compensation as necessary to align physician compensation practices with external reimbursement schemes. As Medicare and other payers increasingly focus on quality, cost management, and related concerns through pay for performance or similar reimbursement tools, an increased emphasis on these measures will occur in physician compensation arrangements.

Consideration of ancillary services

Unlike in a private practice environment that is capable of relying on the Stark Law's in-office ancillary services exception and is therefore able to furnish and permit physicians to receive compensation from ancillary services (for example, imaging technical component, outpatient prescription drugs, and others), the typical IDS will not be structured or operated in a manner to permit direct consideration of ancillaries in determining physician compensation. This is due to the organizational structure used (for example, frequently involving direct employment by a hospital) or the strategic decisions that are made regarding service delivery (such as placing physicians in a captive group practice entity but relocating ancillary services to the hospital because of the higher levels of hospital-based reimbursement that are often available for the same or similar services in a non-hospital setting).

Where the IDS physician organization is a true "group practice" that is separate and apart from the hospital both legally and organizationally, some consideration of ancillary services may be feasible, and a typical "private practice" compensation model is more likely to be available. In most instances, however, more of a type of direct employment model is used (regardless of the particular IDS's legal and organizational structure). As a result, individual physician performance is measured for compensation purposes and ancillary service referrals or utilization may not be considered as part of the compensation plan. In these instances, in order to provide market-competitive compensation, the compensation plan will typically use a percentage of gross professional charges, dollar amount per work or total RVU, or similar measures. In most instances, the defined dollar amount will be linked to market data including that contained in the MGMA and other surveys. Because market data include information from practices that have ancillary services that contribute to physician pay levels, the use of market information arguably provides surrogate credit for physician production in the integrated setting without direct consideration of ancillary service utilization in the IDS.

Performance expectations

An important component of effective compensation plans is the clarification of physician performance expectations. Such expectations should include simple and objectively verifiable measures such as weeks worked per year, days of clinical service per week, on-call obligations, and minimum levels of professional service productivity. More subjective measures, such as participation in group administrative activities, outreach obligations, citizenship, professionalism, quality of care, and related issue areas, may sometimes be defined. Measures that focus on objectively verifiable requirements tend to be easier to administer and more widely accepted by physicians. Subjective measures, which frequently focus on behavior, teamwork, and related issues, usually only apply to a relatively small portion of any physician's total pay.

Other issues

A range of other practical, operational, and other issues are usually addressed in connection with a physician's compensation plan and the physician's underlying employment arrangement. These issues usually include defining processes to address inadequate physician performance through performance improvement plans. The contractual process will usually define performance expectations related to days worked, hours worked, patient visit volumes, and other expectations. In every instance, integrated systems will build on their own experiences — good and bad — with physician relationships in trying to craft compensation and overall relationships with physicians that will meet all parties' needs and goals.

COMPENSATION LEGAL ISSUES

Various legal prohibitions affect physician compensation arrangements. Not surprisingly, the specific legal rules that will affect any particular compensation plan will also be the product of context and, specifically, the nature of the IDS, its structure, and the physician–IDS relationship. Put otherwise, different rules and options relative to compensation will apply depending on whether the IDS involves a for-profit or not-for-profit legal entity; whether the IDS's affiliated physicians are direct employees of a hospital, a captive group practice within the system, or some other component of the system; and other factors.

While the potential range of legal issues is enormous, the primary legal restrictions include the requirements of the federal physician self-referral or Stark Law, the federal anti-kickback statute, and laws and rules applicable to tax-exempt organizations. A general discussion of these laws and rules as applied to physician compensation arrangements follows. Consult Chapter 3 for information on other legal issues that may impact an IDS.

Stark Law

The federal physician self-referral law or Stark Law generally prohibits physicians from making referrals of certain services to organizations with which the physician has a financial relationship. Specifically, under the Stark Law, a physician cannot make a referral to an entity for the furnishing of certain "designated health services" that may be payable by Medicare or Medicaid if the physician (or an immediate family member of the physician) has a financial relationship with the entity, *unless* an exception under the law applies. Claims for designated health services furnished in violation of the law are denied and repayment is required. The law also provides for fines under certain circumstances, and physicians and organizations that violate the Stark Law can also be excluded from participating in the Medicare and Medicaid programs.

Final regulations implementing portions of the Stark Law were published in 2001, 2004, and 2007. The final rules address many important provisions of the law including clarification regarding what services constitute "designated health services." The rules also provide details on many of the law's specific exceptions, including exceptions applicable to the direct employment or contractual relationships between an IDS component and an affiliated physician, as well as compensation arrangements that are permitted to be used when the IDS involves a physician organization that can qualify as a bona fide "group practice" under the Stark Law.

Major implications of the Stark Law and final rule in the context of IDS–affiliated employment and other contractual arrangements include the following:

- **Designated services.** Various services provided by hospitals and medical groups are defined as designated health services and are subject to the Stark Law prohibitions. These include laboratory, radiology and other imaging services, outpatient prescription drugs, and inpatient and outpatient hospital services. Because these services are frequently provided to the patients of hospital-affiliated physicians, a Stark Law exception must be identified and relied upon to allow those physicians to make referrals to various organizations, including the hospitals themselves, for such services.
- **Group practice qualification.** If desired, IDS–affiliated medical groups may be able to qualify as a "group practice" for purposes of the Stark Law. Such a qualification can enable the IDS–affiliated group to provide laboratory, x ray, outpatient prescription drugs, and other designated health services through the group practice and retain revenues from those services to pay group operating expenses, physician compensation, and other costs.

In most instances, an IDS will rely on the Stark Law's exception for employment arrangements to permit the payment of compensation to IDS–affiliated physicians for their services. The core requirements of this exception are that the compensation must be for the physician's personally performed services, consistent with fair market value, and not in any way based on the volume or value of the physician's designated health service referrals. This affects both the amount of compensation that can be paid and the manner in which that compensation is calculated. Importantly, this means that for purposes of measuring physician production and productivity under an IDS compensation plan, where the employment exception to the Stark Law is relied upon, only the work of the physician may be measured and no direct productivity credit may be provided for services furnished by others (for example, no credit may be provided for midlevel production or incident-to services).

Assuming that an IDS–affiliated group qualifies as a group practice for Stark Law purposes, compensation arrangements for group physicians must be structured to comply with the Stark Law and final rule. The result is that the group can furnish designated health services and retain revenues from those clinical laboratory, radiology, outpatient prescription drug, or other designated health services provided through the group. The group could also pool and allocate those revenues (either gross revenues or net of expenses) within the group as part of the group's physician compensation plan. Such a pooling and distribution methodology would be subject to the requirement that the distribution not be based upon the volume or value of the physician's referrals (plus other applicable requirements).

The Stark Law also affects the compensation arrangements with group physicians, regardless of whether the group independently furnishes designated health services (i.e., through the group itself) or whether such services are furnished by the system. Specifically, the Stark Law final rule prohibits the payment of any compensation based on the volume or value of the employed physicians' referrals (or other business generated between the parties). In this instance, the referrals would include referrals for designated health services including inpatient and outpatient hospital services, clinical laboratory services, outpatient prescription drugs, or other services that are defined as designated health services under the Stark Law.

Even if the group's physician compensation arrangements comply with the requirements of the Stark Law, the ultimate level of compensation received by each physician would still be subject to the requirements of reasonableness under applicable tax-exempt organization rules to the extent that all or portions of the IDS are themselves tax-exempt.

Anti-kickback law

A second legal consideration that is applicable to physician compensation arrangements is provided under the federal anti-kickback statute. In general, this law prohibits the payment of any remuneration — essentially anything of value — in exchange for physician referrals.

Specific safe harbor restrictions and statutory exceptions are provided under the anti-kickback law for compensation paid to employed physicians by the

IDS. Other safe harbor provisions are frequently relied upon to allow for other financial transactions such as those used in the medical group (such as medical director agreements). In all cases, hallmarks of a legally compliant compensation relationship include the existence of written agreements (for example, contract documents) governing the contractual relationship, a contractual term of at least one year, the requirement that the level of compensation paid under the agreement is consistent with fair market value, and other more specific requirements.

Tax-exempt issues

Provisions of the Internal Revenue Code (IRC) governing tax-exempt organizations impose restrictions on both the amount of compensation and the methodology used to determine and pay compensation by tax-exempt organizations such as many integrated systems and/or hospitals and their affiliated physician employees and contractors. IRC section 501(c)(3) generally provides that hospitals can receive and maintain tax-exempt status so long as they operate exclusively for religious, charitable, or educational purposes and "no part of the net earnings of which inure to the benefit of any private shareholder or individual." These requirements have been construed to prohibit hospitals from paying excessive compensation to "insiders" including physicians, hospital management, and others. They have further implications for the manner in which compensation is determined and paid — the compensation plan methodology.

Until 1996, organizations that violated the requirements of IRC section 501(c)(3) risked losing their tax-exempt status — although such a drastic remedy was only rarely imposed. In 1996, however, Congress enacted IRC section 4958 — the intermediate sanctions legislation — which provides for an "intermediate" remedy to the revocation of an organization's tax-exempt status. The intermediate sanctions law imposes taxes on persons who are influential to tax-exempt enterprises and who either benefit from or approve transactions that are not consistent with fair market value. Specifically, section 4958 provides for the imposition of personal excise taxes on "disqualified persons" who benefit from "excess benefit transactions." Taxes may also be imposed on the organization managers who approve those transactions. An excess benefit transaction occurs when an exempt organization provides an economic benefit to a disqualified person and receives less than the value of the benefit in return. Transactions that are reasonable and consistent with fair market value will not constitute excess benefit transactions.

Compliance with both IRC sections 501(c)(3) and 4958 requires, as a practical matter, that compensation levels paid to physicians and others in an organization who are deemed to be disqualified persons must be "reasonable" and consistent with fair market value. Compensation is reasonable if it is in an amount that would ordinarily be paid for like services, by like enterprises (including for-profit businesses), under like circumstances. Compensation for this purpose includes all items of compensation including salary, fees, bonuses, severance payments, vested and earned deferred compensation, and other benefits.

In addition to the question of reasonableness, various Internal Revenue Service (IRS) materials give guidance that provides the foundation for the development of acceptable compensation methodologies — ways to determine and pay compensation in the context of an exempt organization. Physicians and other health care professionals are frequently mystified by the changes that are required in compensation plans used by tax-exempt hospitals, as compared to their private practice arrangements. Guidance from the IRS relating to section 501(c)(3) has consistently expressed concern — if not an outright prohibition — on compensation that is based upon a true distribution of net income from the exempt organization (for example, basing physician compensation on true "profits" within the organization).

Because of these provisions, compensation arrangements used with physicians in tax-exempt organizations must be crafted to comply with applicable tax-exempt organization rules and requirements. This is particularly true when net revenues-minus-expense models are used. Given the body of law governing tax-exempt organizations, models that involve a true collection of money by an IDS, payment of overhead, and provision of some or all of what's left over after expenses to physician employees requires close attention to compliance detail. The IRS is interested both in the amount of compensation paid and in how the compensation is determined.

In general, incentive compensation arrangements that have been approved by the IRS tend to include the following safeguards:

- The existence of an arms-length contractual relationship between the tax-exempt organization and the other party (an employee, manager, etc.);
- The assurance that the incentive payments help to promote the exempt organization's charitable mission in furnishing health care services to members of the community;
- The amount of compensation must not be dependent principally upon incoming revenue of the exempt organization, but rather upon the accomplishment of the objectives of the compensation contract;
- A review of actual operating results reveals no evidence of abuse or unwarranted benefits (for example, the compensation that was paid was not unreasonable in amount); and
- The presence of a ceiling or reasonable maximum so as to avoid the possibility of a windfall benefit to the service provider based upon factors bearing no direct relationship to the level of service provided.

In light of these safeguards, various methodological and process protections are typically imposed in compensation plan methodologies to help promote both the reasonableness of compensation levels and the compensation methodology itself. IRS Revenue Procedure 97-13, dealing with tax-exempt bonds, also imposes certain requirements that have been viewed to inform, if not apply directly to, physician compensation arrangements with tax-exempt hospitals and other exempt organizations.

Safe harbor provisions under IRS Revenue Procedure 97-13 impose a number of requirements that, if met, place a compensation transaction within a safe harbor arrangement. Those requirements include:

- The assurance that the amount of compensation is reasonable for the services rendered, with no compensation based in whole or in part on a share of the *net profits* from the operation of the exempt facility; and
- Arrangements that are generally *not* treated as net profits arrangements include the payment of compensation based upon:
  - A percentage of gross or adjusted gross revenues (net of bad debt, adjustments, etc.) or a percentage of expenses from a facility, but not both.
  - A capitation fee or a per-unit fee (for example, one based on RBRVS RVUs). The use of these methodologies in the context of a compensation plan is generally not considered to be based on a share of net profits.
  - Payment of a productivity reward equal to a stated dollar amount based on increases or decreases in gross revenues (or adjusted revenues) and reductions in total expenses — but not both — in any annual period during the term of the contract. Such an arrangement generally does not cause the compensation to be based on a share of net profits.

Not surprisingly, the methodologies discussed in the IRS materials are illustrated in the examples reviewed earlier. It is for this reason that many IDSs use compensation practices that rely on "payer-neutral" measures of physician work or production, such as those involving gross professional service charges, work, or total RVUs. Likewise, RVU-based systems involve a predetermined fee per unit of service, thereby helping to promote the exempt organization's mission in providing services to patients without regard to ability to pay. And while compensation practices that use net revenues-minus-expense methodologies are used, these models require close attention to compliance detail and, as such, tend to comprise a minority of the compensation practices used in IDS today.

CONCLUSION

Physician compensation is an issue that physicians and management have addressed since the inception of organized physician practice. As solo physicians and group practice organizations have gradually migrated to larger, more sophisticated groups and integrated systems, the practice environment has become more complex. As a result, the challenges in developing, implementing, and maintaining effective compensation plans have also become more complex.

The importance of an effective physician compensation plan in an IDS cannot be understated. The experiences of the past demonstrate that poorly designed compensation structures can lead to significant financial losses, unhappy physicians, and a variety of other unintended consequences. In the place of ineffective straight salary or similar arrangements that are disconnected from physician work, we have seen compensation systems that are productivity based and that tend to promote greater physician responsibility and accountability for their own performance and pay levels. More recently, compensation system alignment with the "market" has become more important due to physician shortages and the emergence of a national market for recruitment and retention for many highly sought physician practice specialties.

Moreover, as the external reimbursement environment continues to change, the compensation practices of today and tomorrow will likely still stress the personal performance of the physician, but production will likely continue to expand beyond the classic definition of productivity to also consider cost, quality, and related factors.

External reimbursement will combine with the realities of internal IDS financial management to define what is truly feasible and sustainable in terms of compensation practices. Integrated systems have historically been able to take advantage of differential reimbursement for services in a hospital or physician practice setting. These differences in reimbursement from third-party payers have typically brought more money to the table in an IDS setting, therefore making additional funds available for indigent care, enhanced benefits, recruitment, and physician compensation. The combination of the growth of health care expenditures and significant economic challenges facing the nation may make these historical advantages of the IDS more difficult, if not a thing of the past. If so, the IDS will need to ensure that its compensation and overall financial management systems are sustainable. In the last analysis, physician compensation must be perceived as being fair, yet remain within the limits of market reality and performance.

REFERENCE

1. Medical Group Management Association, *Physician Compensation and Production Survey: 2006 Report Based on 2005 Data* (Englewood, CO: Medical Group Management Association, 2006).

CHAPTER EIGHT

How to Turn Loss into Profit: Addressing IDS Financial Issues

Robert C. Bohlmann, FACMPE, and Kenneth T. Hertz, CMPE

Operating loss attributed to medical practices acquired by hospitals represents a major dilemma among integrated delivery systems (IDSs). It's a complex issue that few have successfully mastered. Medical practice operating loss is an issue that everyone wishes would go away: dealing with it is often pushed back and ignored, but periodically it blasts its way to the forefront. Although IDS leaders may say, "we have to resolve this problem now," the solution is often hard to grasp.

This chapter addresses practice loss by recognizing the many underlying reasons for it. The negative impact on physicians, as well as the IDS, is explained. Most important, the "how-to" or strategy required to productively deal with business realities and resolve practice red ink are explored.

The chapter follows in sequence the practice loss issue along the typical trajectory of reducing or eliminating this loss:

- Perception: Practice loss — is it real?
- Understanding: What is the impact on physicians and the IDS?
- Examination: What are the contributing factors to IDS practice loss?
- Benchmarking: How can you quantify opportunity?
- Resolution: Are there realistic solutions to the problems?

PERCEPTION: PRACTICE LOSS — IS IT REAL?

The majority of primary care medical practices — whether solo, small groups, or large organizations — operate on a close to break-even basis. This trend is now making its way to specialty and multispecialty practices. The usual method of financial management is that money is collected for services rendered, all costs are paid, and what is left is distributed as compensation. Sometimes, limited profit or retained earnings are reported and, frequently, a slight loss is experienced. In the final analysis, continued loss cannot be sustained because physician owners are responsible for capitalization and debt amortization. Most physicians tend to be risk averse in terms of practice investment. Typically, private practice financial statements, and most always tax returns, are reported on a cash basis of accounting.

If we accept this reality in which medical groups break even, why then, do the same practices report losses upon acquisition or integration within a hospital system? The reasons are multi-faceted to the extent that it becomes difficult to comprehensively identify and quantify each component as it is aggregated into a total loss. These losses average $60,000 to $90,000 annually, but can exceed $200,000 per physician per year. The Medical Group Management Association's (MGMA's) *Cost Survey for Multispecialty Practices 2008 Report Based on 2007 Data* reports median loss of $86,181 among the 97 groups reporting, and $75,784 for the primary care groups reporting.[1] It is interesting to observe the extremes among the groups reporting to the survey — a $208,008 median loss among those in the bottom 10 percent, contrasted by a positive $7,997 at the 90th percentile. The mean for all groups responding to the survey is an annual per-physician loss of $97,807.

These reported IDS losses on medical practices are derived from audited financial statements. However, much of this data consists only of revenues and income obtained in the medical practice without credit or consideration of the ancillary revenues the practice produces; in many integrated systems those revenues go into the system instead of the medical group. When medical groups join systems, their providers often perform their ancillary services at the hospital. Those performing ancillary services in their offices find that the income is credited to the IDS instead of the individual provider.

This loss of credit for ancillary revenue runs counter to an important survival strategy for many private groups. A trend over the last several years has been the increased utilization of ancillary services within practices to offset a declining reimbursement base. Given the importance of ancillary revenue to private practice financial viability, it is no wonder that a practice in an IDS will show a loss when ancillary revenue is eliminated from its profit and loss statement. This is not the only contributor to the red ink problem but it is an important component.

Thus, the industry faces a dilemma in arriving at consideration of the "why," "what," and "how" of practice loss. In other words, why is the loss incurred, what part of it is real loss, what is the cost, and how do we arrive at a solution? These questions will be examined in detail in this chapter, but first, attention should be directed to the enormity of the problem as it impacts all aspects of an IDS.

UNDERSTANDING: WHAT IS THE IMPACT ON PHYSICIANS AND THE INTEGRATED DELIVERY SYSTEM?

Historically, operating loss has had significant adverse impact on integrated systems. Attention is directed to events of the last decade. In the 1990s, a surge of practice acquisition by hospital systems took place. At that time, hospitals were also competing with physician practice management companies (PPMCs), such as Phycor, MedPartners, and Promedco, to name a few. Physicians selling their practices to PPMCs and hospitals were typically paid upfront. The phrase, "he who owns the most docs, wins!" seemed to amplify the trend.

By the end of the 1990s, a complete reversal took place, with most PPMCs experiencing financial failures because of the flawed strategy. Within several years, those "darlings of Wall Street" went from high flyers to financial disasters — or at least that seemed to be the attitude of the investors, including physicians who had sold their practices to PPMCs and accepted stock for the perceived value of their practices.

Hospitals also began to take a second look at what they had done. The response across the sector seemed to have four basic elements:

- We are losing money;
- We don't know how to manage or relate to physicians;
- Although we are tied together legally as being integrated, in fact, the pieces of the system are dis-integrated; and
- Our strategy is also flawed!

The result was that many integrated systems terminated (referred to as privatization) their physician component. Physicians ended up "on the street" with limited assets; many were forced to assume a private startup debt that sometimes exceeded $100,000 per physician. And in most cases, this unanticipated transition back to private practice left physicians with ill feelings about their former hospital partner.

This pattern of integration followed by disintegration during the past decade was not the rule, however. Other integrated systems stepped back and, with a thoughtful determination, said, "Yes, there are problems, but strategically, practice integration was the right course of action. We do need to re-engineer, but we intend to stay the course." Many of those systems have retained physician staff; evolved into strong, market-dominant organizations; and, thereby, benefited from a determined long-term strategy. Yet, many of them still wrestle with practice loss or reported losses.

As health care approaches the end of the 2000 decade, the integration trend, which reignited in 2005, has reached epidemic proportions in some areas of the United States. There is a sense in many communities that integration was a correct strategy in the first place but the organizational concepts were flawed. With those mistakes behind them, many integrated systems seem to have declared: "this time we'll get it right!"

These statements withstanding, "getting it right" leaves most IDSs still grappling with the issue of financial loss. Until the dilemma is fully understood, it is likely that the decisions that led to unfortunate organizational unraveling in the 1990s may continue to be made.

Financial loss is the problem that won't go away. It frequently resurfaces on the agendas of IDS chief executive officers (CEOs) and boards, first, as an annoyance but then escalating to priority status. The impact of these losses resonates across systems, adversely impacting physicians and their support staff in many ways.

Physician responses to this demon can be summarized as feelings of being a drag on the system because they require financial support. This is combined with the physicians' feelings that they are not getting their proper credit for total funds flow dollars. This is certainly not the attitude that creates an enthusiastic partnership. Poor morale does not encourage positive patient service. Thus, all stakeholders have a stake in resolving these issues.

Further, when physicians are told to reduce the loss, it is often stated in a large unquantifiable sum that no one can get their hands around. Conversely, a defined level of responsibility, specifically oriented to a physician practice, typically represents an achievable objective.

The concern over attribution of significant loss related to integrated practices is a cloud hovering over a very strategic segment of any IDS, affecting not only physicians but all segments of the organization. Thus, understanding the full details of what contributes to loss should be identified as a major operational objective as this concern persists.

EXAMINATION: WHAT ARE THE CONTRIBUTING FACTORS TO PRACTICE LOSS?

The first step in the clarification process is identifying and understanding the source and degree of loss. The range and scale of these losses can be staggering. Although the impact and types of losses may differ significantly from one IDS to another, the purpose of this chapter is to accomplish full identification. In doing so, the analysis must be in the context that the point of reference, or definition of loss, is that which is reported in contrast to pre-acquisition performance. In other words, ask *what* is now different? If past financial data is unavailable, assume that breakeven will be the logical point of reference. Years of IDS responses to MGMA surveys indicate that reaching breakeven is indeed possible.

Comprehensive analysis suggests that financial loss can be placed into four broad categories:

- Losses resulting from change in ownership;
- Losses resulting from an accounting system that either includes or excludes the revenue and expense categories reflected within a medical group's practice financial reporting system;
- The impact and influence of policies, decisions, and actions that benefit the IDS but would not be typically applied to the classic medical group; and
- Behavioral changes among physicians who transition from shareholders in an entrepreneurial private practice to employment by an IDS.

If the definition of loss is, indeed, an acceptable point of reference — and, if not, what is — an operating statement line-item comparison to published

MGMA benchmarks represents the scientific approach. In this respect, several references can apply, including MGMA's Cost Survey for both Single and Multispecialty Groups,[1,2] *Physician Compensation and Production Survey,*[3] and the *Performance and Practices of Successful Medical Groups,* also called the "Gold Book."[4] Familiarity with these references is helpful, particularly understanding the terms used (such as "total gross charges," "total medical revenue after operating cost," etc.) because applying the wrong metric can lead to incorrect conclusions, which further complicates the loss question.

Losses resulting from change in ownership

Certain activities take place as a private practice is integrated into an IDS under an employment model. The previous physician practice is terminated and physicians transition as W2 employees or a different organizational status, which may vary depending upon state regulations dealing with corporate practice of medicine. Usually, the physicians making this transition are still responsible for collecting their former practice's outstanding accounts receivable, paying of outstanding accounts payable, and meeting obligations they have made to the practice's stockholders. Debt, if any, may be absorbed by the acquiring system. Fixed assets, including equipment and any separately owned clinic facilities, may also be acquired, leased, or entirely excluded from the purchase.

Specific points of reference contributing to loss within the change-of-ownership category include a delay in revenue (or cash flow), changes in salary and benefits for support staff, and amortization of the purchase cost of the practice.

Revenue, or cash flow

Delay is to be anticipated because physicians practicing under a new tax identification (ID) number must be re-credentialed and a new revenue cycle initiated. Transition to a new practice management system is frequently an accompanying factor in the loss. In some cases, such as when a large medical group is assimilated by the IDS, it will retain its practice management system. Due to the time required for credentialing and computer conversion, it may take more than six months for the physicians' collections to achieve an acceptable level following their transition. This category unto itself can result in a first year loss exceeding $100,000 per physician because operating costs, including physician compensation, begin on day one.

Not only is there a delayed revenue cycle, but the collection process for medical practices is different than for the hospital or IDS. It is not uncommon to encounter an extended learning curve for the IDS to adopt the private practice's style and manner of collection, or vice versa, during the first year following integration of the practice into the IDS.

Salary and benefit change

Many physicians identify continued employment of their support staff as a condition of integration. Many hospitals assimilate practice staff but at an institutional salary level, which can be greater than that paid in private practice. In other words, the employees are integrated at a salary level comparable to that which exists within the system; this can result in a substantial windfall in salary for the practice's staff. Benefits are also likely to vary and, in many cases, increase substantially. Because staff payroll represents the largest cost category in most practices (25 to 30 percent of gross income), the effect on the practice could represent as much as a $30,000 increase equivalency per physician. The cost is one that continues in perpetuity.

Amortization of practice purchase cost

In some cases, the acquisition amortization, or interest, applicable to practice integration is charged back to that unit. Again, this is a cost that would not be incurred by the former private practice.

Losses attributed to accounting system

Integrated systems classically apply hospital accounting systems to their integrated practices. These systems may or may not recognize (add or subtract) revenue and cost line items such as ancillary revenue and indirect general and administrative overhead.

Ancillary revenue

Gross revenue attributed to imaging, lab, and other departments may range anywhere from $50,000 per physician in smaller primary care practices up to levels exceeding $300,000 for multispecialty practices. This revenue, adjusted for collections and assignment of both direct and indirect cost, may contribute as much as $100,000 per physician or as little as $20,000 in the case of a smaller primary care practice that operates only basic radiology and limited laboratory services.

The pre-integration practice financials would typically have included revenue from ancillary services distributed in a fashion meeting compliance requirements. In the IDS, neither the practice nor the individual physicians typically receive credit on the financial statements for "down-stream" revenue generated. Comparing pre- and post-integration financials, the post-integration financial statements typically omit the ancillary revenue, thereby reducing the practice profitability on paper.

Indirect general and administrative overhead

Indirect general and administrative (G&A) overhead can be a factor of consequence and should be recognized when addressing ancillary departments. Even when the hospital system will allocate department profit to the practice, the contribution is usually less because indirect overhead will have been charged by the ancillary department. In private practice, the major contribution of some departments may be limited strictly to assumption of indirect overhead.

The system's indirect G&A overhead is, by policy, charged to the practice department. This category usually includes expenses that are not found in a private practice situation, such as:

- Compensation for the IDS's CEO and chief financial officer (CFO);
- Human resources management;

- Central executive office expense;
- System purchasing; and
- System information technology cost.

Private practices tend to operate with fewer management staff as opposed to hospitals. Thus, an additional administrative G&A burden allocated by a hospital methodology can be anywhere from 2 to 5 percent of gross income even when little direct benefit is added to the practice itself. The system, on the other hand, should benefit in many ways through the addition the of the practice. These additional costs, not present in the pre-integration, further contribute to the stated "loss" by the practice.

Losses attributed to system convenience

Upon or following integration, many integrated systems seek to apply policy or improvements that the acquired practice would not otherwise have needed or applied had ownership remained with physicians. These include:

- **Cost of time lost attributed to heavy meeting obligations.** Although seemingly trivial, this can apply to a commitment on the part of both physicians as well as support staff. Hospitals tend to operate via committees. What is the salary cost of time lost attributed to two or three hours per week per physician?
- **Take all patients.** As mission-based organizations, integrated systems tend to be more limited with respect to aggressively managing payer mix, which results in reduced income. A difference of approximately 1 percent (average mean), as reported in MGMA's Cost Survey, between integrated and private practices does not seem to be significant, but it may represent a $5,000 annual revenue reduction per physician.
- **Relocation or upgraded facilities.** Hospital construction costs are usually higher per square foot in comparison to private practice space. Once acquired, a practice may be a candidate for an upgrade or facelift of its current facility, or a move to a new or more convenient location. These relocations may benefit the IDS or, at least, improve its image, but this is not always a decision that a private practice would have made. While resulting increase in costs of moving a practice facility contributes to the expense side of the ledger, it typically does not generate additional revenue for the practice.
- **Additional departments that benefit the IDS.** For example, one organization became interested in tracking system referral so it created a department to pursue this objective and hired a manager and information technology support staff. This department added nothing whatsoever to the practice's bottom line, but did benefit the system. What it also did was add a cost of approximately $3,500 per physician to the practice overhead.
- **Electronic medical record (EMR).** EMR application in private practices is still limited because of economic limitations; however, electronic systems do represent a core requirement in most hospital practices. The additional costs for the deployment of the EMR are added to the practice's cost basis in the post-integration financial statements, which further contributes to the imbalance of the profit and loss statement.

Losses associated with a change in physician practice style driven by the new financial model provided by the IDS

This last category is one for which the physician can, or should, accept more responsibility. Compensation based on productivity represents a major point of contention, or opportunity. It is related to the strategic objectives adopted by the IDS.

Early in the 1990s, integrated systems offered physicians significant guarantees based on their earnings while in private practice as recruitment inducements. Promises within these documents were made without any correlation to the physician's continued productivity. In the absence of incentives, it was common to see these physicians' patient volumes decrease. Not only did they see fewer patients, but also they frequently reduced their schedule of hours and weeks worked. Vacations, which were rarely taken in private practice, became the routine with hospital employment.

Even where incentive compensation plans were in place, integrated practices became a haven for physicians who wished to work part-time or on reduced schedules with a quality-of-life objective. It is difficult to dispute these personal objectives, but an economic reality still existed where full-time resources were required to support a practice. In some cases, revenue may not have been much greater than the level of support costs and, thereby, contributed little or nothing to cover providers' salaries and expenses. The problem vexing organizations today is that more members of today's generation of practicing physicians favor working in large groups with more part-time work arrangements. Supporting this trend is the fact that half of today's medical school classes is female. As mentioned in Chapter 1, it is common for female physicians raising young families to seek such part-time work arrangements for part or all of their careers.

Physician compensation based on work units, versus what is left over as margin dollars, have become the stated affiliation objective for physicians in many private practices with heavy Medicare/Medicaid payer mixes. Hospital-based physicians today typically are compensated on productivity systems, usually related to work relative value units (RVUs). These compensation systems are established on the basis of a strategic decision on which the system has executed an integrated practice. To turn around and hold a profit hammer over physicians thus employed negates or does not acknowledge the system's basic strategic concept.

In addition, physicians who transition to an IDS tend to lose their entrepreneurial spirit if not credited for the work they perform. This credit helps create a cost containment philosophy within a private practice. Without it, it is easy for physicians to adapt to a mode of behavior philosophy of requesting convenient overhead support, such as an extra employee or additional examining rooms. Control of or realistic responsibility for support costs should be acknowledged as being within a physician-controlled domain. Either this is exercised by administrative decree or adopted within the physicians' incentive compensation program, as discussed in Chapter 7.

BENCHMARKING: HOW CAN YOU QUANTIFY OPPORTUNITY?

The process of identifying and analyzing the multiplicity of factors that influence revenue, cost, or operating loss is applied to benchmarking as a management engineering technique. This methodology creates an identification opportunity, as well as quantifies the degree of opportunity. Opportunity degree, in turn, provides a basis for establishing priority within a well-orchestrated financial turnaround project. Thus, analysis can occur in a logical sequence. Exhibit 8.1 identifies some key benchmark reference points for a medical practice operated by physicians compared to hospital operations.

As previously noted in this chapter, definition clarification is the critical basis to applying and interpreting comparative data. For example, charge and revenue information can be misleading. Revenue for MGMA Cost Survey comparison purposes represents cash collections, but in an accrual-based hospital system revenue usually is identified as charges. The difference between cash collections and charges can be substantial.

A second and equally important point applies to charges and collections per physician. For the purposes of the MGMA Cost Survey, whether reporting on a practice specialty or multispecialty basis, this reference includes all revenue categories *in addition to* professional services. These categories will include ancillary services and midlevel, non-physician providers. On the other hand, the MGMA *Physician Compensation and Production Survey* charge and collection benchmarks are related to professional services only as the basis. It should be noted that a few limited survey applications do include additional revenue, but these are the exception.

Exhibit 8.1 also illustrates the type of information that can be interpreted when assessing the various components of an IDS operation. These line items are just a few of the many indicators available.

If "why is the practice losing money?" is the question, then the response is to compare the IDS practice with the financial performance of private, or physician-owned, practices. Exhibit 8.1 shows how this is done. For example, gross charges among integrated systems average approximately $390,000 less (or 61.1 percent lower) compared with the private multispecialty group. Some $193,000 of the total differential between IDS and private multispecialty group providers' gross charges is attributed to lab, x-ray, and non-procedural charges. It can, therefore, be concluded that at least half of the gross income differential is explained by the inclusion of nonprofessional charges in the private physician's gross. In comparison, most IDS practices do not receive credit for ancillary services, which is typically the case in private practices. It is assumed that physician ordering habits remain the same irrespective of practice ownership.

Additional observations about Exhibit 8.1 include:

- Comparative physician productivity differential within the IDS category indicates:
  - A range from a 14 percent loss (professional charges), 8 percent (work units), and 12 percent (encounters); and
  - IDS physicians produce less across several categories, including professional charges (–14 percent), work units (–8 percent), and encounters (–12 percent).

EXHIBIT 8.1 ■ Median Value per Physician

	Multispecialty (Not Hospital- or IDS-owned)	Multispecialty (Hospital- or IDS-owned)	Actual Percentage Differential
Total Gross Charges	$1,157,947	$ 766,343	(33.9%)
Total Medical Revenue	$ 718,074	$ 483,625	(32.6%)
Laboratory/Pathology Charges	$ 117,805	$ 49,748	(57.8%)
Radiology/Imaging Charges	$ 107,327	$ 23,507	(78.1%)
Non-Procedural Charges	$ 98,685	$ 57,126	(42.2%)
Medical Professional Charges (Inside)	$ 488,295	$ 419,755	(14%)
Medical Professional Charges (Outside)	$ 82,301	$ 72,663	(11.1%)
Total RVUs	12,211	10,169	(16.7%)
Work RVUs	5,771	5,293	(8.3%)
Encounters	4,929	4,344	(11.9%)
Total Procedures	12,086	8,819	(27%)
Total Operating Cost (Excluding NPP)	$ 435,667	$ 338,649	(22.3%)
Provider Cost			
Non-Physician (Salary/Benefit)	$ 22,461	$ 20,799	(7.4%)
Physician (Salary/Benefit)	$ 257,468	$ 243,861	(5.3%)
Net Income/Loss Excluding Financial Support	**$ 1,487**	**<–$68,831>**	

NPP — non-physician provider
RVU — relative value unit

- The differential in medical revenue (collections) is 1 percent of the differential in charges;
- Operating cost among the IDS is approximately $100,000 less than private practices but represents 70 percent of collected revenue (Private practices operate, per calculation, at 60 percent. The benefit of incremental income is, thereby, illustrated. In other words, when practices have been integrated, resulting in contribution of ancillary revenue to the hospital or system rather than the practice's direct bottom line, there will be a negative impact on the profit and loss statement of the practice.);
- IDS provider cost (physician compensation and benefits) as the major cost item for the practice is within 5 percent of private practice, yet professional

productivity, applying inside services, is 14 percent less (This differential in physician productivity further contributes to the negative nature of the practice's profit and loss statement.); and

- Operating loss resulting from a combination of reallocating ancillary revenue to another department and lower physician productivity results in a negative differential to the integrated practice of close to $70,000.

The conclusion that can be drawn from these fundamental analyses is that two of the major contributing factors to IDS loss are the non-recognition of combined traditional ancillary services ($193,000) plus the negative productivity differential ($78,000). The negative impact to the practice is a total of $271,000, or 71 percent of the $391,000 total charge differential.

An IDS benchmark analysis should not ignore the other revenue/cost categories addressed in this chapter. On a case-by-case basis, there can be considerable differences with revenue cycle limitations frequently being another major area. It is noteworthy that the more obvious areas of consideration stand out, but relatively less significant categories can also be of consequence.

As a caveat to those unfamiliar with MGMA surveys, it should be noted that reporting is on a line-item basis, thus, the categories do not necessarily total. This is due to the fact that participation among reporting groups is subject to wide variance on a line-item-by-line-item basis. The number of organizations reporting is also noted within the survey.

RESOLUTION: ARE THERE REALISTIC SOLUTIONS TO THE PROBLEMS?

Information consolidation represents the first step in resolving the alleged loss issue. The term "alleged" is used because if IDS management states, "we have a loss," the question must be asked, "a loss compared to what and is it really a loss?" Is there a problem, or is loss really the result of accounting transference and/or subjecting a classic physician practice to an institutional environment governed by different ideology? If an IDS financial statement is benchmarked against private practice, it may be apparent operational cannibalization has taken place. To ignore this basic position of clarification begs the question.

Once facts are known, it becomes incumbent upon management to sort through the information and determine which is relative to the initial points identified in this chapter, including:

- The impact of initiating a new business line (the practice). If the impact is increased cash flow attributed to initiating new billing identification and payer credentialing, the IDS has developed an asset in its accounts receivable.
- Costs attributed to physician salary levels. If cost attributed to salary levels is recognized for the offset, then the potential of establishing separate wage/salary levels compared to the private practice may avoid the problem.
- The impact of instituting a new methodology. If the IDS has made changes or instituted new methodology to benefit the IDS as a whole, this should also be recognized.

- Costs attributed to support staff. Support staff salary and benefits represent the major practice cost category, and it is the one where physicians can be influential.

Physician productivity related to performance against benchmarks then realistically pinpoints true loss from an operating standpoint. The first area represents physician, or provider, performance as measured by dollars, patient/hospital encounters, surgical cases, work RVUs, or a combination thereof.

Originally, in the physician practice purchases of the 1990s, many compensation arrangements did little to incentivize physician performance. To the contrary, many employment contracts offered qualities that supported a more relaxed lifestyle. Today, incentive arrangements are most common. Incentives most usually include productivity provisions as the basic compensation contributor. More recently, other incentive measurements include quality, patient satisfaction, access, cost control, and citizenship.

Resource utilization represents the second major area over which a physician may exercise control. When not faced with ownership responsibility, physician motivation may move toward requesting resources that may make practice life easier or facilitate personal productivity irrespective of economic justification. Again, understanding the bottom-line impact of adding additional resources is critical and can be measured through benchmarking.

It is not unusual for a "one size fits all" mentality to prevail in many integrated systems, meaning that resource support is equal for each physician irrespective of patient or case volume. Application of volume-based measurements is extremely valuable in the assessment of reasonable resource application levels. It is particularly helpful when addressing the costs of clinical and clinical support staffing.

CONCLUSION

Identification, classification, and understanding represent the major points of emphasis when addressing practice loss. Responsibility acceptance on the part of executive management and IDS board of directors determines whether practice loss, as a philosophical issue, can be rationalized and accepted. Acceptance of reality should be viewed within perspective of the strategic objective on which concepts of integration are based, as well as those of each individual organization. The value of physician practices on an IDS depends on that system's broad or limited point of reference. This determination is based on both data from the system's financial information system and how that data is interpreted, the goals and philosophy of leadership, and the short and long-term goals of the system.

In the case where the "loss issue" cannot be rationalized by all levels of the organization (from the board to the operating management), then, in fact, the IDS will, in all probability, operate under a dark cloud of ongoing irrational finger pointing. Conversely, those systems who grasp reality and can assign appropriate responsibility should achieve their strategic objectives attributed to integration.

To summarize, key actions to take to understand and then address in IDS loss are:

- Understand the origin;
- Quantify the impact;
- Direct opportunity improvement with the appropriate parties;
- Avoid placing unjustifiable blame on physicians;
- Recognize the total funds flow; and
- Develop overall perspective within the context of the strategic contribution to the total IDS and its realistic opportunity potential.

REFERENCES

1. Medical Group Management Association, *Cost Survey for Multispecialty Practices: 2008 Report Based on 2007 Data* (Englewood, CO: Medical Group Management Association, 2008).

2. Medical Group Management Association, *Cost Survey for Single-Specialty Practices: 2008 Report Based on 2007 Data* (Englewood, CO: Medical Group Management Association, 2008).

3. Medical Group Management Association, *Physician Compensation and Production Survey. 2008 Report Based on 2007 Data* (Englewood, CO: Medical Group Management Association, 2008).

4. Medical Group Management Association, *Performance and Practices of Successful Medical Groups: 2008 Report Based on 2007 Data* (Englewood, CO: Medical Group Management Association, 2008).

CHAPTER NINE

Operational Issues

Cynthia L. Dunn, RN, FACMPE; Nick A. Fabrizio, PhD, FACMPE, FACHE; and Rosemarie Nelson, MS

Among the most difficult decisions in managing an integrated delivery system (IDS) is deciding which corporate operating principles and procedures must be adopted by all of the individual groups within the IDS. This leads to asking how quickly the integration will take place and in what stages. In this chapter, we discuss the key operational issues that go into these decisions.

IDENTITY

If the IDS has more than one hospital, the IDS's leadership must determine whether the IDS should develop a common brand or try to maintain their individuality. While each option has its strengths and weaknesses, maintaining separate identities for these units may result in more limitations for patients and providers if maintaining separate identities results in less effective coordination of care through medical systems, patient transports, information technology (IT), and coverage.

In addition, if one of the hospitals or medical groups is perceived as having a higher quality of care than the others, that institution's leaders may have concerns about being associated with other institutions in the IDS perceived as having a lower level of quality or service. The issues of identity must be resolved because allowing a hospital or group practice to operate in a silo of superiority will prevent it and the other groups, hospitals, and other parts of the integrated system from moving forward with true integration.

VALUE OF A UNIFORM APPROACH

An IDS with 10 separate medical group practices and 10 separate methodologies to process patients is not an IDS. In an integrated system, each practice may have minor deviations, such as hours of operation, compensation arrangements, and physician-to-staff ratios, but other processes — appointment scheduling, check-in, co-payment collection, follow-up on outstanding bills, use of clinical care guidelines — should be uniform to take advantage of the potential synergies that integration can create. This uniformity in major processes also provides a solid framework for the IDS to orient and train staff at all of its owned or managed practices.

Centralized governance of seemingly simple shared functions such as patient registration is essential to developing uniform processes within the IDS that will identify/indicate the singularity of that organization to patients. Centralizing patient registration, sharing processes and rules, and merging infrastructure, such as insurance tables in a common registration system, are examples of the depth of discussion an IDS governing body must be willing to undertake. Complete integration moves to the sharing of appointment scheduling (a referring provider actually makes a patient appointment on the imaging calendar), problem lists, and reconciled medication lists — all of which are key factors to delivering value and safety throughout the IDS.

The IDS must also determine which of its processes will be organized into a "systems" approach to take advantage of market opportunities and create efficiencies. Other factors relate to which organizations will maintain their independence and for how long. Exhibit 9.1 lists some of the areas that need to be addressed in determining whether standards can be achieved in creating operating efficiencies.

PRACTICE MANAGEMENT SYSTEMS

One of the most frustrating issues in integrating hospitals and medical groups is the electronic practice management system. Hospitals and medical groups have long enjoyed having separate practice management systems — each finding systems on the market targeted to their unique needs. Vendors have concentrated on creating these systems as stand-alone entities. While it is possible to find practice management systems that link hospitals or medical groups almost seamlessly, few if any products are designed to link hospitals and medical groups with each other. Few practice management systems integrate anything beyond demographic data — both clinical and non-clinical — from the hospital to the medical group and vice-versa. Only a few vendors offer products that link both the hospital and medical group environments.

One advantage that smaller integrated health systems have over larger systems is that IT integration takes place on a smaller, more manageable scale. For example, a hospital integrating with two smaller medical practices naturally has fewer practice management system users and processes between the entities. Among the disadvantages this smaller IDS faces is that its resources for technology are usually limited. The smaller IDS may also find that vendors are less willing to take the time and effort to customize their solutions to meet the needs of a smaller system.

While large hospitals and health systems that integrate with medical groups can offer more human and financial resources and can spread costs out throughout a larger system, the scale of this endeavor makes integration of technology much more difficult. It often requires the vendor to work with several hospitals and medical groups to create interfacing programs. In doing

EXHIBIT 9.1 ■ The Systems Approach

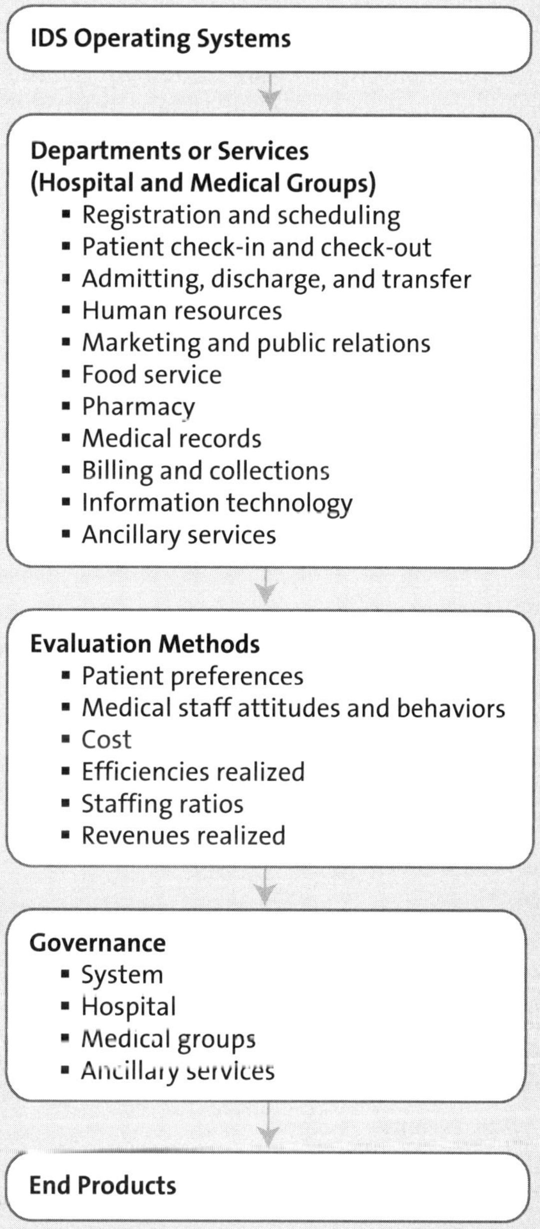
IDS Operating Systems
Departments or Services
(Hospital and Medical Groups)
▪ Registration and scheduling
▪ Patient check-in and check-out
▪ Admitting, discharge, and transfer
▪ Human resources
▪ Marketing and public relations
▪ Food service
▪ Pharmacy
▪ Medical records
▪ Billing and collections
▪ Information technology
▪ Ancillary services
Evaluation Methods
▪ Patient preferences
▪ Medical staff attitudes and behaviors
▪ Cost
▪ Efficiencies realized
▪ Staffing ratios
▪ Revenues realized
Governance
▪ System
▪ Hospital
▪ Medical groups
▪ Ancillary services
End Products

IDS — integrated delivery system
© 2009 Nick A. Fabrizio, PhD, FACMPE, FACHE

so, the vendor must be willing to create effective and ongoing relationships with, perhaps, dozens of separate organizations in the system, and with several other vendors, including some who may be competitors. The challenge facing large integrated systems is that their hospitals and medical groups often have separate IT systems that must be linked together, but only one IT department to work with several vendors to coordinate data interfaces and make the exchange of medical information as seamless as possible.

GETTING PHYSICIAN COMMITMENT TO INTEGRATION

Successful operations require leadership to understand the differences between physician practices and hospital departments. Physician practices cannot be successfully managed as another hospital department is managed. Expertise in the management of physician groups is a requirement. The development and planning of an overall medical practice strategy must address what services will be offered, where they are offered, how long it will take to implement, what it will cost, and what kind of return is expected. IDS leadership should obtain buy-in from those physicians who will help the organization achieve all goals. Leaders must involve those physicians from the beginning of the strategy development.

Integrated systems that perform better than the average exhibit a few common themes: setting realistic goals, obtaining real physician commitment, and managing according to a formal plan. Financial performance expectations are communicated clearly and early in the relationship and are monitored monthly.

TEAM FOCUS ON INTEGRATION OF OPERATIONS

The IDS must assemble an operations team that can work with IT professionals from both the hospital and medical group environments. This team should examine the several key integration activities that are important to successfully integrate patient care with and between the various medical groups, clinics, hospital(s), and other components of the IDS.

Key integration activities include:

- Connecting providers with hospitals and medical groups in real time;
- Allowing for the safe and compliant transmission of medical information to and from all locations;
- Connecting patients to the hospital and medical groups;
- Connecting the hospital(s) and the medical groups together via information systems;
- Allowing for advanced electronic services for patients (such as the ability to request and schedule appointments, inquire about and pay bills, ask providers questions, request prescription refills, etc.);
- Generating useful management reports for both the hospital and medical groups (such as census reports, relative value units [RVUs], encounters, charges, collections, accounts receivable management, case mix, physician quality reporting initiative [PQRI], etc.);
- Providing patients with medical information and education; and
- Creating dashboard indicators to monitor the health of the system — for patients, providers, and management.

EFFICIENCY: THROUGHPUT

A critical task for any IDS is to analyze the parts or departments and offices of the IDS that affect patient care from the clinical departments to the back-end office functions including the billing department. Often, medical centers and practices focus on patient *throughput*, or the time it takes a patient to complete each task between appointment scheduling and check-out. It is important for medical practices to eliminate the inefficiencies from process to process in the medical practice. Eliminating inefficiencies may not only help to make the office more efficient, but also it may decrease costs and improve patient satisfaction. A measurement of process efficiency should include the time that patients wait in the reception area and at all other points along the encounter flow.

Some organizations also analyze throughput as it relates to patients trying to access their hospital or medical practice; for example, calling the practice and spending time waiting on-hold. Others measure throughput by how long it takes for referring providers to get their patients seen by a specialist or how long it takes the operating room to process patients or get patients scheduled in operating room block times.

Capturing information about throughput is a time-consuming task. Fortunately, several electronic health record (EHR) systems are able to capture blocks of time between patient stops throughout clinical areas or departments, whether they are in the medical group or the hospital. EHRs are able to time-stamp every action, capturing and calculating the information in real time. Electronic systems also make reporting the results easier. When possible, collecting data through the practice management system or EHR is preferred.

If electronic technology is not available or is incapable of tracking throughput time, managers are advised to measure time by using the throughput tracking grid shown in Exhibit 9.2. Before starting this time–motion study, practices or departments should determine the duration of the survey and the sample size needed to draw conclusions. The organization's leadership team will need to give thought to how many human resources (time, mainly) it wants to devote to data collection, how the information is to be collected, the duration of the study, and how to process the results.

By analyzing information collected in a time–motion study through a tool like the one shown in Exhibit 9.2, practices or departments can better understand where the bottlenecks are in their department. They can then form project teams to understand the causes of variation and develop improvement strategies to streamline operations and improve efficiencies.

MULTI-SITE MANAGEMENT

Managing practices in multiple sites presents an additional challenge because the parent organization must work to standardize the policies and processes between the different entities and minimize or eliminate duplicative services or multiple systems including the practice management and electronic medical record (EMR).

EXHIBIT 9.2 ■ Throughput Tracking Grid

XYZ Department

Provider name: ______________________

Date: ______________________

Appointment type: ______________________

Steps	**Time**
Appointment time	
Patient arrival	
Chart pull-up	
Roomed for provider	
Provider enters exam room	
Provider exits exam room	
Provider enters exam room	
Provider exits exam room	
XR/Lab in	
XR/Lab out	
Check out	

The role of scale

As discussed in Chapter 5, the goal of achieving and leveraging the scale or size of one's organization is to create an effective management structure that fosters collaboration among the medical groups and hospitals. Hospitals can be structured by service line, matrix, functions, or divisional design. Integrating the physician practices into whichever organizational reporting structure is present is vital to success. However, more important than the structure or design selected is the effective and efficient coordination of activities between the medical groups and the hospital. Attaining this coordination achieves integration.

Critical to satisfying and accomplishing the objectives of integration is an operations committee. The committee's membership should be broad enough to encompass a representative sampling of key stakeholders from the medical groups and hospitals. The operations committee must also give its members the authority to resolve issues or act as the conduit to reporting problems to higher authorities and then resolving those issues in a timely fashion. Having a working operations committee will help the organization bridge the gap between the policies, procedures, strategies, and results of the individual departments and how those parts relate to the whole. This will help the IDS better

EXHIBIT 9.3 ■ **Scale of the IDS**

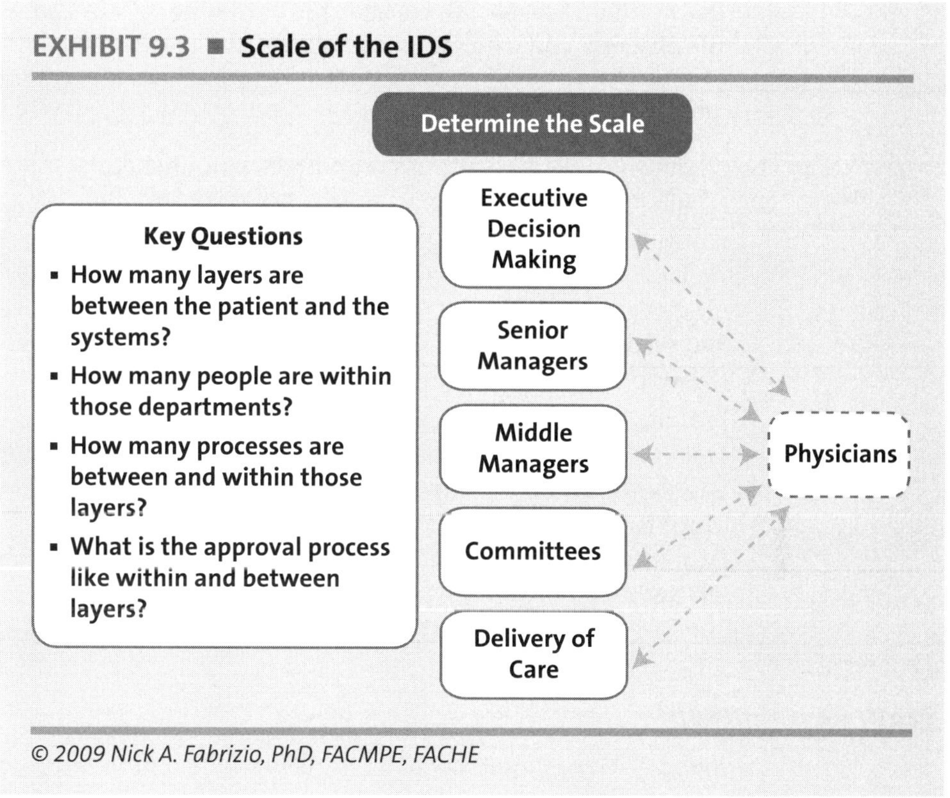

© 2009 Nick A. Fabrizio, PhD, FACMPE, FACHE

understand the scale of the organization and how many steps and reporting levels exist between the patients and the providers or the delivery of service.

One of the key steps in determining scale is to also look at the entire organization and all of its parts and determine how care is delivered. This examination includes getting an understanding of how many steps and reporting levels there are between IDS decision making and patient care. Once the operations committee understands these issues, it should prioritize them and make recommendations to an executive-level committee. This executive body should be made up of system leaders including physician and non-physician leaders. Some of these leaders should be representatives of the respective parts of the IDS. Exhibit 9.3 is an example of the processes that must be analyzed when looking at the scale of the IDS.

Operations committee

Establishing operations committees in an IDS facilitates the communication of information about activities at ground zero (where patient care is delivered) to the executive committee or board responsible for the overall financial health of the organization. One of the early challenges in forming an operations committee is to identify key participants from the various clinics to serve on the committee. Members should be limited to those office/department managers who are knowledgeable in their department's operations and skilled in representing the physician's concerns. The operations committee's main task is to analyze the operations from the clinic level and to report problems and recommend solutions to those on executive leadership committees. This committee will be vital in collecting and disseminating information and implementing process improvement strategies. When possible, the operations committee should also have physician representation as well as clinic directors or service line managers.

The functions of the operations committee could include:

- Establish performance measures and indicators that would be reported monthly or quarterly as dashboard indicators or key process indicators (KPIs);
- Implement strategic and operational support for physician recruitment and retention initiatives;
- Develop clinic budgets and business plan development;
- Evaluate and propose new ventures;
- Manage cost and overhead management;
- Work with the physician representatives to develop processes to deal with disruptive physician behaviors; and
- Establish and monitor an effective patient referral process between hospitals and to and from physician practices.

THE REVENUE CYCLE PROCESS

Team development

Integrated systems should consider implementing a process-centered revenue cycle. A process-centered revenue cycle will enable all of the practices, clinics, and other sub-units of the IDS to have a unified, seamless payment process with clear lines of accountability to achieve target outcomes. In this type of management model, revenue-cycle functions that are usually fragmented among different departments are coordinated in an outcomes-driven payment process with clear accountability and performance measurements.

A process-centered revenue cycle model contains three principal components:

- The core process is configured around delivering one set of payment outcomes (rather than the by-product of collected departmental primary and secondary activities); outcomes are improved if one entity is responsible for leading and directing the activities throughout the other sites;
- The process is integrated from start to finish, from both provider and patient perspectives; and
- The entire process is supported by coordinated operational and financial information and performance measurement.

From the patient perspective, all steps — creating an account, scheduling an appointment, receiving and paying a bill — are viewed as a seamless, coordinated process. For individual practice managers and staff, the process-centered revenue cycle is constructed as a single process with a series of essential steps, all with clear downstream effects and impact on payment outcomes. Front-end staff (for example, registration and admitting personnel) view collection of patient demographic and insurance information as the primary means to ensure appropriate payment for services. Back-end staff (for example, the billing office) see claim denials as indicators of process breakdowns and the motivation for education and corrective action.

In the process-centered revenue cycle, what are usually considered separate functions are linked through prescribed communication mechanisms, standardized policies and procedures, common results reporting, and performance measures. As front-end and back-end staff and providers are linked, they begin to function as a team, singularly focused on achieving improved revenue-cycle outcomes.

When assessing the revenue cycle process and practice management system at each medical practice, it is important to think about maximizing revenues and controlling and minimizing costs and work. Focus on process, technology, and personnel:

- **Process.** Do the current systems have built-in reconciliation and workflow management to keep all employees accountable and proactive?
- **Technology.** How do supervisory personnel deal with vendors, secure backups, and critical incidents like network outages or disk crashes? How do they manage the current personnel? Are available tools deployed for optimal outcomes and effective utilization?
- **Personnel.** What is the knowledge level of workers? What are their credentials? How frequently is training provided? Are they capable of independent problem solving?

Credentialing

Credentialing, according to Wikipedia (www.wikipedia.org), is defined as the administrative process for validating the qualifications of licensed professionals, organizational members, or organizations. Most hospital systems assign this procedure to the medical staff office. In an IDS the responsibility could fall to a risk manager; in many cases this manager may be the best suited individual on staff to coordinate the credentialing process. The risk manager works in tandem with the business office, communicating the status of each physician in the credentialing process. Proper and timely credentialing is essential to receiving payment from insurance companies; in some instances this process could take up to six months. Therefore, credentialing should be initiated early and completed before the provider begins seeing patients.

All physicians who join the IDS will have to be recredentialed with each insurance company before proper payment can be initiated and completed. To help manage this process the Coalition for Affordable Quality Healthcare (CAQH) has created the Universal Credentialing Datasource. This free service simplifies and improves the credentialing process for physicians and other health care providers. With Universal Credentialing Datasource, provider information is entered one time — online or by fax — to satisfy the credentialing and recredentialing applications of all participating health plans, hospitals, and other managed care organizations. Updates can be made instantly, and encryption technology keeps all data safe. Many insurance companies now require providers to have a CAQH application on file before they will credential or recredential a provider.

Fee schedules

Establishing a suitable/useful fee schedule is challenging. Revenue generation for a medical practice is based on one simple question: "Are its fees competitive?"

Analyzing what the various practices charge for their services is a basic financial review tool that will allow the practice to stay competitive in the market.

Often, the analysis of practice fees is performed soon after the practice is purchased by the IDS. As for most analyses, the analysis of practice fees begins with a benchmark comparison. An accepted benchmark is the Medicare Fee Schedule. Using the Medicare Fee Schedule provides several advantages. It applies nationally and is used by many health care providers as the basis for analysis or comparison. It is updated regularly and adjusted for regional differences in wages and cost of living.

When analyzing practice fees, gather the following information from each medical practice:

- A copy of its current fee schedule (the schedule should list all procedure codes that are billed with a corresponding charge);
- A copy of the current Medicare Physician Fee Schedule from the Centers for Medicare & Medicaid Services (CMS); and
- A report from the past 12 months (minimum of 6 months) listing all billed procedures, number of times each procedure billed, and the collected amount.

An example of a fee analysis spreadsheet comparing a practice's fees as a percent of Medicare and as a percent of a payer is shown in Exhibit 9.4.

A fee schedule analysis should be performed annually as part of the financial planning for the medical practices. It verifies that the practices' coding is current and accurate and that they have competitively priced procedures.

EXHIBIT 9.4 ■ Coding Frequency Chart

CPT Code	Description	Frequency	Medicare Allowed Amount	Your Current Fee	Your Fee as a % of Medicare	Health Plan Payment Rate	Health Plan Payment as a % of Medicare
99203	Level 3 office visit, new patient	385	$ 94.18	$115	122%	$105	111%
99213	Level 3 office visit, established patient	2269	$ 51.63	$ 65	126%	$ 58	112%
99232	Subsequent hospital care	596	$ 54.27	$ 65	120%	$ 60	111%
99214	Level 4 office visit, established patient	1977	$ 80.65	$100	124%	$ 90	112%
45330	Sigmoidoscopy	112	$117.28	$125	107%	$125	107%
93000	Electrocardiogram	198	$ 25.76	$ 50	194%	$ 45	175%
99396	Preventive visit, established patient	211	$104.27	$130	125%	$105	101%
81002	Urinalysis	588	$ 0.00	$ 12		$ 5	

CENTRAL BILLING OFFICE

Accounts receivable management touches many parts of the hospital and its affiliated physician network. Success is best accomplished by engaging various "stakeholders" in the billing process, from office staff to providers. When assessing the billing office functions of the individual medical practices, consider the following process steps:

- Forming a work group, including staff from the IDS central billing office, central administrative office including the financial officer, and representatives from selected practice sites;
- Documenting the current structure and performance;
- Creating a transition plan to move to central processing;
- Establishing performance and accountability standards; and
- Creating a communications and training matrix.

A centralized billing system shares its billing rules across all providers and specialties. Therefore, errors discovered and corrected for one provider will be avoided in the future for all of the providers using the system.

Provider-based billing

Physician or clinic services furnished in a nonprovider setting (for example, a traditional free-standing clinic location) are generally reimbursed by Medicare under the Medicare Physician Fee Schedule with a single, global rate. Those same services furnished in a provider-based setting are reimbursed in two separate components:

- The hospital facility payment under the ambulatory payment classification (APC) rate for the outpatient hospital services; and
- A separate payment for physician services under the Medicare Physician Fee Schedule, reduced for the hospital site-of-service.

The combination of the APC payment and the reduced fee schedule amount can be substantially greater than the global fee schedule payment for traditional free-standing clinics. Primary care practices with relatively high Medicare utilization such as internal medicine and family medicine should consider provider-based billing as an option.

Provider-based billing has advantages and disadvantages to consider. Advantages of provider-based billing include:

- The opportunity for increased reimbursement for services furnished to Medicare beneficiaries (in some cases, increased payments of 50 percent or more can be realized); and
- Access to hospital resources that may not be available otherwise (including sharing of hospital information services, quality assurance, compliance, purchasing, managed care contracting, and human resource functions).

Disadvantages of provider-based billing include:

- The extent to which changes are necessary in order to implement the new billing process (the extent of change depends on the degree to which the current operations are already integrated with the main provider, such as the hospital); and
- The reactions of patients to receiving care at a provider-based location instead of at an alternative provider that is not provider-based. This can be measured by patient-satisfaction surveys.

There are many provider-based regulations and requirements that need to be considered. CMS issued final rules for implementing the prospective payment system for outpatient hospital services several times during the past several years with final clarification of its policies in Program Memorandum A-03-030 published on April 18, 2003.

An area that should be reviewed before switching to provider-based billing is the distinction between the requirements for on-campus and off-campus sites. CMS defines *campus,* in part, as "the physical area immediately adjacent to the provider's main buildings, other areas and structures that is not strictly contiguous to the main buildings but is located within 250 yards of the main buildings, and any other areas determined on an individual case basis, by the CMS regional office, to be part of the provider's campus."

Exhibit 9.5 lists the essential requirements for all medical practice locations. (Note that off-campus sites must also satisfy all of the requirements applicable to on-campus locations.)

One issue that causes confusion for patients when a medical practice changes to provider-based billing relates to financial liability. If a change is made, all Medicare beneficiaries must receive written notice before the delivery of services of the amount of the beneficiary's potential financial liability for coinsurance on both the professional service and the hospital outpatient visit. If the exact type of service is unknown, CMS will allow the hospital to furnish a written notice to the patient that explains that he or she will incur a coinsurance liability that would not be incurred if the location were not provider-based. This may discourage Medicare beneficiaries from obtaining care at a provider-based location if care can be received from an alternative provider that is not provider-based.

Before making a decision to change to provider-based billing, follow these process steps:

1. Perform a detailed reimbursement analysis to determine the potential financial impact of changing to provider-based reimbursement. (Note that the change in reimbursement only applies to Medicare outpatient services currently performed in the location[s] being considered for provider-based status.)
2. Form a work team to closely review the provider-based requirements and obligations applicable to each location.
3. Develop a list of unmet requirements and identify barriers and the changes that would be necessary to meet the provider-based requirements.

EXHIBIT 9.5 ■ Provider-based Facility Checklist*

√	Critical Requirement (all must be met)	
	Licensure: Provider-based departments must be operated under the same licensure as the main provider, except in areas where the state requires a separate license for the site.	
	Clinical Integration: The clinical services of the provider-based department or entity are integrated with the main provider (hospital) and are treated as any other department of the hospital with respect to the following areas:	
		Hospital privileges of the professional staff
		Monitoring and management oversight
		Reporting by the medical director
		Responsibility for medical activities such as utilization review and quality assurance
		Medical records
		Access to inpatient and outpatient services of the main provider (hospital)
	Financial Integration: The financial operations of the provider-based department or entity are integrated within the financial system of the main provider (hospital) as evidenced, for example, by a complete sharing of income and expenses, as well as common accounting and reporting of financial data.	
	Public Awareness: The provider-based location portrays itself as being part of the main provider (hospital) such that patients entering the department are aware that they are entering the hospital and will be billed accordingly.	
	Compliance:	
		Complies with the Emergency Medical Treatment and Active Labor Act (EMTALA) requirements as amended by the Centers for Medicare & Medicaid Services (CMS) on September 9, 2003.
		Physician services furnished in the hospital-based department are properly billed with the correct site-of-service indicator so that the Medicare site-of-service payment reduction for physician services can be properly applied.
		Complies with all the terms of the hospital's Medicare provider agreement and physicians comply with Medicare's nondiscrimination provisions.
		All Medicare patients are hospital outpatients for billing purposes. Medicare payments for services in a hospital-based department are subject to the 72-hour payment window provisions applicable to prospective payment system (PPS) hospitals.
		Applicable hospital health and safety rules for Medicare-participating hospital-based departments are being met.
	Ownership and Control: The provider-based department or entity is owned 100 percent by the main provider (hospital) and must be under the direct control of the hospital.	
	Administration and Supervision: The reporting relationship between the provider-based department or entity and the main provider (hospital) has the same frequency, intensity, and level of accountability that exists with any other hospital department. Administrative functions, such as billing services, human resources, payroll, and purchasing services, are handled by the same personnel for both the hospital and the provider-based site.	
	Location: The provider-based location is within 35 miles of the main campus of the hospital, or it is demonstrated that the hospital and the provider-based department share a common service area.	

* Additional requirements could apply, obtaining the advice of counsel and other advisors is recommended.

4. Estimate the cost to the organization of complying with each requirement.
5. Identify the qualitative aspects of transitioning to a provider-based location, such as the public perception of increasing costs to Medicare beneficiaries.
6. Compare the advantages and disadvantages of provider-based status and make a decision on whether or not to proceed with provider-based status in each location.
7. Formulate an action plan to achieve provider-based status, if applicable.

CONTRACTING

Key performance indicators, also known as KPIs, help an organization define and measure progress toward organizational goals. Once the IDS has analyzed its mission, identified all of its stakeholders, and defined its goals, it needs a way to measure progress toward those goals. KPIs are those measurements. They are quantifiable measurements, agreed to beforehand, that reflect the critical success factors of the IDS. These indicators, listed in Exhibit 9.6, are for specific units or offices and the IDS entity as a whole.

EXHIBIT 9.6 ■ Key Performance Indicators

1. **Service volume (varies by specialty)**
   a. Based on the procedure codes, how many billable services are provided?
   b. What is the mix of services? By specialty, a percent by codes billed, or by patient?
   c. What is the charge entry process? (List the number of steps and staff positions involved.)
   d. What is the lag time for charges entered with respect to the date of service?
2. **Has the staff been trained to:**
   a. Effectively (accurately and quickly) enter the data?
   b. Be familiar with insurances (such as the order of primary and secondary insurance coverage)?
   c. Identify the responsible party for the claim (such as workers' compensation, auto insurance, grants, etc.) to ensure that the bill is sent in a timely manner?
   d. Verify information for the carrier?
3. **Practice fees**
   a. How often is the fee schedule reviewed?
4. **Prepare an audit**
   a. Identify the top 10 to 30 codes via an explanation of benefits (EOB) from a sample of payers. Do the allowances equal the fees?
5. **Coding**
   a. Have the codes and/or levels of codes that are billed been adjusted to allow lower or no reimbursement?
6. **Payer makeup**
   a. What is the payer mix (Medicare, Medicaid, managed care, workers' compensation, self pay, etc.) based on charges for your top 5 to 10 payers during the past 12 months?
   b. Has your payer mix shifted toward payers with lower allowance schedules?
7. **Adjustments**
   a. How often are adjustments made on accounts?
   b. Who gives write-off approval?
   c. Is the adjustment policy in writing and what is the monetary limit?
   d. Have the contractual adjustments been validated?

CONCLUSION

There are several considerations an IDS must address related to operating successful entities such as medical practices. One of the most important factors that leads to inefficiencies is the multiple processes that individual medical practice offices bring to the IDS. Certainly, each practice would like to maintain their best practices; however, the IDS must determine which of these processes are unique to that office or group and should be maintained, and which process can be standardized to gain efficiency and economies of scale.

CHAPTER TEN

Information Technology in the Integrated Delivery System

Cynthia L. Dunn, RN, FACMPE, and Rosemarie Nelson, MS

TECHNOLOGY IMPLEMENTATION IN AN INTEGRATED DELIVERY SYSTEM

The demand for sophisticated business intelligence reporting and clinical automation has increased throughout the health care industry. Many hospitals, laboratories, and ancillary testing centers have initiated connectivity services for physicians to access patient information. Exhibit 10.1 illustrates the depth of interconnectedness and layers of functionality affecting a health care community.

As integrated delivery systems (IDSs) expand, they seek to harness the power of new technology to improve both financial and clinical performance. The array of increasingly sophisticated information technology (IT) needs will require a strategic and systematic approach to system acquisition and implementation in integrated health care delivery systems.

IT strategy within an IDS must address a variety of users. In addition to IDS–owned physician practices, IT solutions encompass ancillaries, hospital inpatient and outpatient operations, and private physician medical groups affiliated with the IDS. An enterprise approach facilitates the exchange of patient information to more effectively coordinate care. A master patient index is an example of one mechanism within an IDS IT solution that provides fluid sharing of patient information across entities within the IDS.

Of course, each IDS is as unique as each practice within that community. A multi-hospital IDS with several campus sites and hundreds of employed physicians that represent only a percentage of the community will have different resources and strategies as compared to a small IDS that has one Critical Access Hospital and the majority of community physicians employed by the IDS. In either extreme, the defining orientation in the development of an IT strategy is based on the dominant partner in the delivery system: the hospital or the physician community.

EXHIBIT 10.1 ■ **Health Information Network**

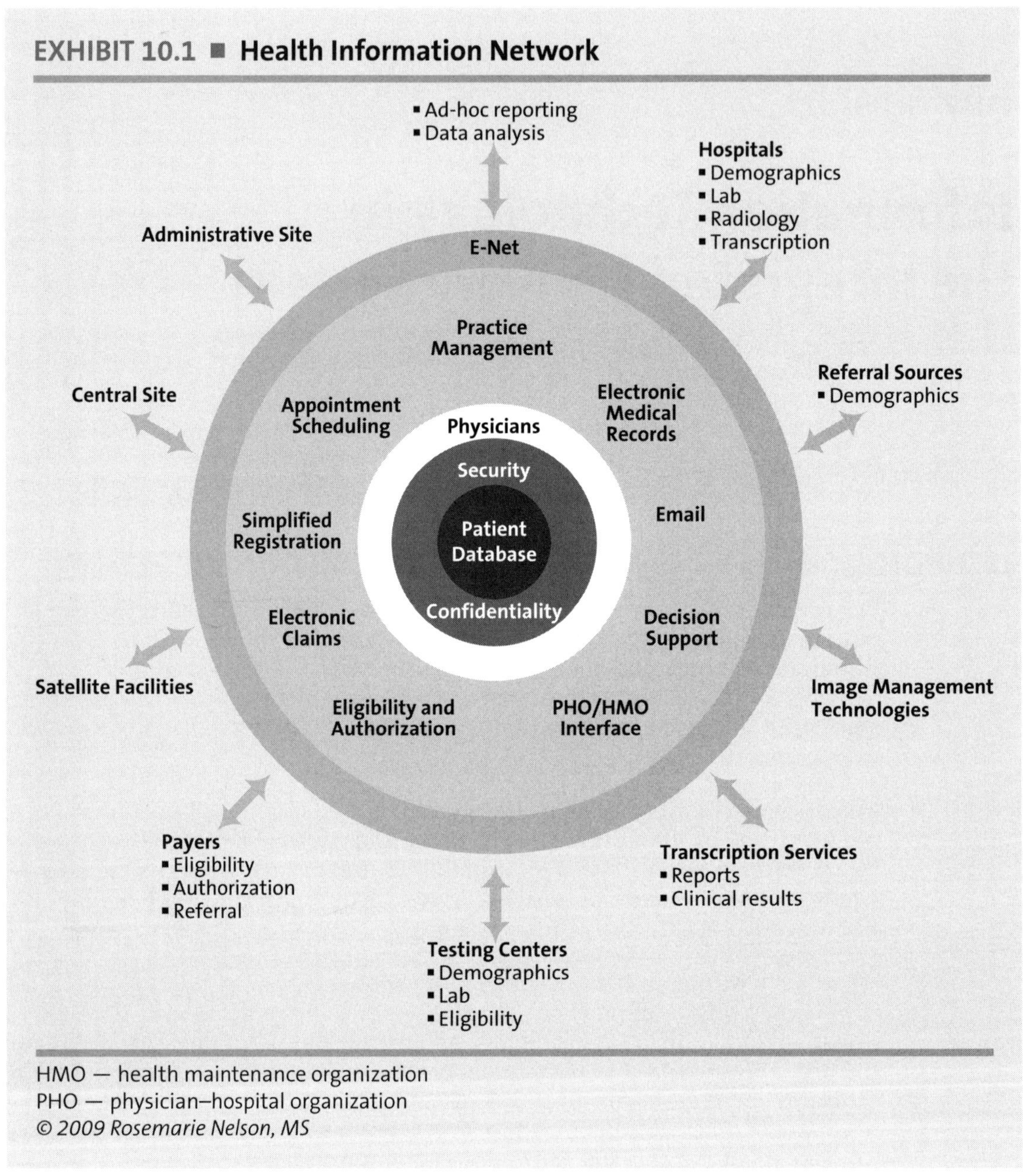

HMO — health maintenance organization
PHO — physician–hospital organization
© 2009 Rosemarie Nelson, MS

The physician practice that is committed to partnering with a hospital-led IDS may find the IT environment of the hospital less amenable to solutions aimed directly at physician practices. The risk to the practice is implementing a solution that meets the needs of the IDS but does not optimize day-to-day operations for the physician practice.

For example, when implementing new technology into the hospital(s) and physician practice(s) in an IDS, such as an electronic health record (EHR), it is essential to determine the key requirements and functionality of the technology before moving forward in the process. A unilateral decision may result

Calculating ROI for an information technology purchase

Direct equipment cost

___ Purchase price
+ ___ Finance costs
+ ___ Facility modifications
= ___ Direct equipment cost
___ Years for payback
___ Annual utilization

Direct equipment cost ÷ years for payment and utilization = Direct equipment cost per procedure per year

Supply and utility cost

___ Annual supply cost
+ ___ Annual utility cost
= ___ Annual supply and utility cost
___ Annual utilization

Annual supply and utility cost ÷ utilization = Supply and utility cost per procedure per year

Direct labor cost

Step 1. Estimate staff labor cost

___ Average salary per full-time-equivalent (FTE) employee
+ ___ Benefits
= ___ Labor cost per FTE

Step 2. Estimate staff time for equipment

___ FTE to operate equipment
___ Annual utilization

Labor cost per FTE × FTE to operate ÷ by annual utilization = Labor cost per procedure per year

Cost savings

___ Cost of previous technology or process
+ ___ Labor cost for positions eliminated
= ___ Cost savings per year

Cost savings per year ÷ annual utilization = Cost savings per procedure per year

Training costs

___ Initial training cost (first year)
___ Time period for payback

Initial training cost ÷ time period for payback

= ___ Amortized initial training cost
+ ___ Annual training cost after first year
= ___ Annual training cost

Cost savings ÷ annual utilization = Annual training cost per procedure per year

Revenue from increased productivity

___ Increased provider procedures (e.g., office visits, surgical procedures)
___ Revenue per procedure

Increased provider procedures × revenue = Total revenue from increased productivity per procedure

Annual revenue to practice

___ Direct equipment cost per procedure
+ ___ Supply and utility cost per procedure
+ ___ Labor cost per procedure
− ___ Cost savings per procedure
− ___ Annual training cost per procedure
+ ___ Revenue per procedure
= ___ Net revenue per procedure

Net revenue per procedure × utilization = Annual net revenue

___ Annual net revenue
+ ___ Total revenue from increased productivity
= ___ Annual revenue to practice

Adapted with permission from D. N. Gans, "Calculating ROI for an information technology purchase." *MGMA Connexion*, Vol. 5, Issue 4, April 2005.

in dissatisfaction and undermine the benefits of adding the new technology. Hospital and physician representatives must undertake a joint discussion about their vision of patient care with the technology implementation. Issues to be reviewed and discussed include:

- Current systems in use;
- Ownership of data;
- Recoupment of investments made to date;

- Changes in workflow;
- Data standards; and
- Interoperability.

The IT plan is the core of a strategic and systematic approach to system acquisition and implementation. The plan must be developed within the context of the organization's strategic goals and objectives. Reaching these goals and objectives requires a *data strategy* that identifies the organization's plans to build a data infrastructure and the use of data standards. The *migration and implementation strategy* describes the sequencing of projects including infrastructure and application acquisition and implementation and organizational change. That migration strategy positions the organization for incremental acquisition of best-of-breed applications or for a phased integrated solution implementation across entities (inpatient, outpatient, medical practices, ancillary services, etc.).

HOSPITAL AND GROUP INTEGRATION STRATEGIES

Connectivity within an IDS may be as simple as dictating the application of choice for all users, or as complex and sophisticated as the need to develop interfaces to several systems. The challenge of connectivity is heightened when attempting to bring together several practice management systems and physician practice electronic medical records (EMRs) along with systems for:

- Laboratory information;
- Radiology information;
- Materials management;
- Surgery scheduling;
- Patient admission, discharge, and transfer; and
- Billing and collections.

And then there are the many systems for other ancillaries as well as medical equipment such as electrocardiographs, bone densitometers, blood analyzers, and video-based scopes with their own proprietary digital output.

The key consideration in a selection project begins with defining needs and the objectives to be gained with the implementation of the technology. From the definition of those goals, the benchmarks are created against which systems can be measured during the selection phase. The scope of the project explicitly states what is to be achieved and why. The scope must be clearly defined, understood, and agreed upon. Clearly stated, the goals establish the basis for the implementation phase.

Start with defining requirements by documenting the processes (flow charts) and obtaining feedback from key stakeholders. Consider setting short (< 6 months), medium (6 to 12 months), and long (> 12 months) term goals, with measurable targets to help assess your progress toward those project goals. Goals need to be realistic, attainable, and communicated to all, as well as take into account the current and future infrastructure of the IDS and each practice within the system. Because of this, goal-setting should take place on two levels: an IDS–centric level and a practice-specific level, which means each practice participates in a goal-setting exercise. Those practice-specific goals are rolled up into the IDS umbrella plan.

THE SELECTION PHASE

The old saying, "they all look the same to me," often comes to mind when one sits down to view system demonstrations. However, as one moves forward through the process of selecting technology, it becomes apparent that this is not the case. Many systems offer similar functions and features, which makes selecting the right system to meet the needs of an IDS difficult and somewhat daunting. To avoid distractions of the bells and whistles that many systems offer, keep the following definition foremost in your mind as you go through the selection and implementation processes:

> Technology is a tool to optimize operational efficiency and provide high quality care and service to patients via a user interface for providers and staff that improves job satisfaction.

It is likely that the hospital component of the IDS has an established system in place that supports the inpatient clinical operations including pharmacy, lab, imaging, and physician orders. Although the vendor supporting that clinical information solution may also provide a solution directed at the outpatient, ambulatory environment, it is not necessarily the optimal solution and should be considered as one option in the selection process. The best-of-breed approach —finding the best product for each function, even if from different vendors — may be preferred when considering how best to meet the goals and objectives established in the early planning phase. Interfaced best-of-breed products are a viable alternative to seeking an integrated solution from a single vendor.

Where to start

Information systems and information management are keys to the organization and its development. IT can be compared to the body's central nervous system that carries messages back and forth among providers, administrators, and staff performing the tasks and services. The conduit in an IDS provides the mechanism for referral relationships and improved quality of care to patients seen within multiple entities in the IDS.

The first step is to create a multidisciplinary team that includes representatives from registration and reception, medical records, billing, clinical support (medical assistants or nursing), medical secretaries, providers, and IDS administrative support. The team should also include IT staff that span the variety of entities within the IDS. For example, at least one primary care provider and one specialty provider should be included on the team along with other team members representing the variety of IDS departments and practices in place. The team will need a project coordinator or leader to drive the process. Several projects have stalled because the team was led by a physician champion who continued to have full-time responsibilities in the care of patients.

Management skills that include delegation, coaching, and monitoring are all necessary as the team steps through goal-setting, practice readiness, product research, request for proposal (RFP) determination, budget development, system scoring, and vendor proposal evaluation. The most successful implementations are led by professional managers, many of whom have a clinical background (lab analysts, nursing informatics, etc.) and are partnered with a physician champion. IT involvement and support are critical, but this is not an IT project; it is a quality initiative with a strong focus on operational improvement.

Focus on goals and objectives, not software bells and whistles

An introspective approach is necessary to establish the goals and objectives for the technology implementation. Survey all prospective users at all the clinic sites with the following three questions:

1. What is your objective to be achieved with the implementation of the technology? (What is/are the problem(s) you are trying to resolve?)
2. What is your preferred solution to automating the process at issue?
3. What must the new tool do/provide for you to be willing to use it?

As discussions around these questions evolve, it is important to manage expectations. For example, it is unrealistic to expect that an EHR will improve visit documentation while the staff devotes less time to recordkeeping — those are contradictory goals, and it is unreasonable to expect a better product outcome with less effort.

The first step for the team is to articulate the goals. Goal writing is not simply an academic exercise; goals drive the selection and specify the implementation plan. For example, an ineffective goal is "improve productivity." A goal that specifies how to achieve improved productivity is "ability to re-issue prescriptions directly with pharmacies to free up nurse time for in-clinic patient activities."

The project team can simultaneously assess the readiness for the EHR. Mapping workflow and assessing physician and staff members' computer skills (see Exhibit 10.2) are specific tasks to identify the issues that will match to functionality.

The mapping-of-workflow exercise must be completed on two levels: the global IDS level in terms of interactions and transactions between the IDS departments and the ambulatory practice settings, and in the individual practice setting with the clinical operations of the practice. Analyzing each step, which user performs each process, and the cycle time involved will provide insight to how each technology product will fit the practice and how the practice will improve operationally by re-engineering each process.

Certified systems

One of the areas of concern is the lack of technological standards in the EHR marketplace. As a savvy and knowledgeable business you understand the

EXHIBIT 10.2 ■ Employee Skills Checklist

Basic computer skills are the foundation on which further computer knowledge is based. To help with training preparation, please complete the following questions as honestly as possible. Use the following rating system:

1 = Inexperienced
2 = Slightly experienced
3 = Fairly experienced
4 = Very experienced

Experience Level	**Yes/No**
Have you ever had any formal computer training?	
	Rating
How would you rate yourself as a computer user, in general?	
List any practice management systems you have experience with and rate your experience:	
Please rate your experience with the following programs:	
Microsoft® Word	
Microsoft® Excel	
Microsoft® Outlook	
Internet Explorer	
Skill Assessment	
Turn on a computer, monitor, and printer	
Properly shut down a computer	
Adjust the monitor	
Use a mouse for controlling the cursor	
Use a keyboard for controlling the cursor	
Start a program by double-clicking an icon	
Start a program from a program list or Windows display	
Find and respond to screen prompts	
Start up Internet Explorer or Netscape	
Navigate between programs and tasks	
Demonstrate familiarity with the layout of the standard keyboard	
Locate the up/down arrows, delete key, back-slash key	
Create a word file, write a document, and save the file/document to a disk or e-mail the document	
Use the keyboard commands or the mouse to highlight text; delete, cut, copy and paste text; make the text bold or change the font size	
Spell-check a document	

(Exhibit continues on next page)

EXHIBIT 10.2 ■ Employee Skills Checklist *(continued)*

Skill Assessment	Rating
Retrieve a word file and save changes made to it	
Print a Microsoft Word, text, or .rtf document	
Use Print Preview and send a document to a printer	
Use Print Preview to view a document before printing	
Print a document; knows difference between hard and soft copy	
Select menu items from a drop-down menu	
Demonstrate an understanding of page orientation for document layout	
Consider what needs to be printed (for example, number of pages to print)	
Send an attachment via an e-mail message	
Select or change the printer	
Start an application and create a document	
Name and save a document in an appropriate folder or directory	
Retrieve, revise, and rename a document	
Demonstrate an understanding of the difference between "save" and "save as"	
Demonstrate an understanding of various peripherals, such as a portable drive or a pen drive, Bluetooth, and infra-red	
Demonstrate an understanding of and use dialogue boxes	
Demonstrate an understanding of the general structure of an e-mail address	
Interpret features of an inbox (for example, the owner, date, subject, and size of an e-mail message)	
Interpret features of a new message (for example, To, Cc, and Subject)	
Interpret features of a retrieved message (for example, From, Date sent, Reply, and Forward)	
Retrieve and reply to an e-mail message	
Forward an e-mail message	

importance of making your selection based upon accepted industry standards. An organization that has created a certification program is the Certification Commission for Healthcare Information Technology (CCHIT). CCHIT is an independent, nonprofit, public–private organization that sets the benchmark for health care IT.

The certification process is based on real-life medical scenarios designed to test products against the clinical needs of providers and the quality and safety needs of health care consumers and payers. CCHIT works in collaboration with several other organizations to regulate standards, develop prototypes for national health information network architecture, and assess privacy and security laws and practices.

CCHIT certification has limitations. For example, some of the interoperability criteria have not been created, and some specialty-specific software cannot

The CCHIT Certification Criteria

The CCHIT certification process tests and inspects products on a comprehensive set of criteria for:

- **Functionality** (the ability to create and manage electronic records and automate workflow in a physician's office)
- **Interoperability** (the ability to receive and send electronic data to other entities such as laboratories)
  - The software must be able to receive and transmit information in six (6) categories:
    - Laboratory and imaging;
    - Medications;
    - Immunizations;
    - Clinical documentation;
    - Secondary uses of clinical data; and
    - Administrative and financial data.
- **Privacy and security** (the ability to keep patients' information safe)
  - The software must meet criteria in four (4) security categories:
    - Access control;
    - Audit;
    - Authentication; and
    - Technical services
  - And in three (3) reliability categories:
    - Backup/recovery;
    - Documentation; and
    - Technical services.

be certified. Some critics of the process feel the certification standards are too broad, allowing many of the vendors a fairly straightforward path to certification. Other objections are based on specific, mandated criteria perceived to raise the costs of products in the market.

CCHIT certification is one element of testing a vendor's commitment to the marketplace. Certification is modality-, version-, and year-specific. As this text was written, CCHIT criteria and work groups exist in the areas of ambulatory EHR, inpatient EHR, emergency department EHR, electronic prescribing, health information exchange (HIE), interoperability, security, and personal health records (PHR). To date, CCHIT has added new requirements each year, so the 2009 certifications may not satisfy the 2010 requirements, for example. In addition, certification is version-specific. This, along with the high cost of applying, may make vendors wait until their latest version is released before seeking certification.

How to make the selection "cut"

It is not unusual to identify 10 to 15 different products at first blush. However, it will be necessary to narrow the list to four or five products for the demonstration stage of the selection process. Start by visiting the vendor's Website and view online demonstrations of the product. Visit trade shows and see what types of organizations are visiting the vendor's booth (existing clients and prospective clients) — are they similar to your organization or are they vastly different in size or mix? Network with peers and listen to what people say about the products you are considering. Search the Web for articles or case studies including references to those products and try to determine if the organizations profiled in the studies are similar to your system. It may be beneficial to engage a reputable consultant who is familiar with a wide range of products to assist with this specific phase.

A request for proposal (RFP) or request for quote (RFQ) adds discipline to the selection process. The RFP sections typically describe the purpose and general information for the project. Include background information about your organization along with project objectives to enable the vendor to appropriately quote a solution. The application and hardware requirements along with training, maintenance, and installation services should also be requested. Of course the projected costs, any unspecified requirements, and vendor references are additional key components.

The total cost of ownership includes *soft* and *hard costs*. The new system — hardware and software — is a hard cost. Implementation and training costs are examples of soft costs. The vendor's response to the RFQ should include both types of costs. Each entity must prepare a network readiness assessment, business process analysis, staffing assessment, conversion plan cost projections, and an estimate of revenue reductions or delays in reimbursement. The ongoing costs for maintenance will grow as the number of user licenses and workstations increases.

How do you know it can work?

The demonstration evaluation and reference site visits are the tangible tests for how effectively the product can meet pre-determined goals and objectives. It is important to script the vendor demonstration to focus on the desired outcome of the implementation. Discuss how processes will change with the implementation. For example, do physicians issue verbal orders? How will that be accommodated in the automated environment? See the flow of results and how they are approved and processed electronically. Understand how existing paper processes will change post-implementation. Score the demonstrations with a written tool and simple scoring.

Always de-brief with those attending the demonstration immediately after it is completed. You may have to ask the vendor to leave the room for the

15 minutes it will take because you do not want to lose the physicians or nurses attending to patient care duties.

Vendor contract review

A contract from the vendor will be written from the perspective of the vendor organization. Take the time to review the contract and request changes in language that you find objectionable. Specifically:

- Look at the warranty, disclaimer, and limitation of liability sections;
- Review the indemnification section;
- Read the duration and termination clauses — the organization should have an easy "out" with relatively little organizational pain;
- Understand the different ways in which the vendor can terminate the agreement and make a contingency plan for this; and
- Resist the temptation to take shortcuts to save money on training. Training is often the first place organizations try to save money — don't! Add a vendor re-visit three months after the go-live date to help determine what features and functions are underutilized.

Absolutely engage an attorney experienced in software contracting to assist with the final step in your selection process.

Building relationships with vendors changes the rules of engagement. The need for solutions versus commodities is at the core of the changing environment. Technology is a dynamic field, and the vendors are a source of information as IDS leaders often find it impossible to remain current with the constant market changes and offerings.

Educate the vendor on your needs, preferences, decision-making process, and people involved. Realistically set expectations for vendors during the sales process because it will help set the stage for ongoing support and service (see Exhibit 10.3). A few old clichés are worth remembering:

- There is no free lunch.
- Health care organizations that look for "deals" may find they have found problems.

Contracts are critical documents that are important to buyers and sellers. The best contract is one that is mutual, reflecting a "win-win" result.

IMPLEMENTATION AND TRAINING

As you think about adding a technology solution, keep the end in mind. With a fully implemented solution, what do you expect your operation to look like? How do you see user interaction with the technology in day-to-day flow? The technology is a tool, not the end result. Re-engineering of some work processes will be required, and planning for these changes must occur for a successful outcome. It is essential to facilitate change in processes and eliminate manual functions and manual analysis of data.

EXHIBIT 10.3 ■ Questions to Ask Technology Vendors

To manage technology vendors effectively, an organization should:	What to ask the potential vendor partner:
▪ Appreciate the value of various technology investments and their cost/ benefit ratio.	▪ What are the equipment requirements? ▪ Does the application require the latest gadget and a state-of-the-art computer replaced every year?
▪ Understand that systems are dynamic and need to be constantly aligned with changing conditions.	▪ How do you approach "down time," when no problems or questions are coming in? ▪ How do you stay engaged with customers to anticipate needs and application of technology solutions?
▪ Be dedicated to training all staff to keep technology and operations aligned.	▪ What's your approach to disseminating technology on an ongoing basis? ▪ How do you manage that process?
▪ Employ a multidisciplinary approach to strategic information systems and IT decision making.	▪ How do you include non-technical staff in a technical process to achieve buy-in and enthusiasm for the adoption of new technology?
▪ Maintain clear accountability for the multitude of tasks and activities involved in systems and technology management.	▪ How do you manage urgent requests while maintaining progress on longer-term projects?

IT — information technology
© 2009 Rosemarie Nelson, MS

Discuss the concept of change management within your organization. Introducing major change into any workplace can create stress and confusion and lead to other, unanticipated changes. A health care organization — large or small — is no exception, and introducing new technologies such as an EHR requires significant change.

Can your organization make the transition? Can your staff, including the nurses, understand and manage the process? Has the impact of the change been discussed throughout the organization so that everyone has a clear understanding of its impact on their personal futures? Employees often fear technology will replace them and perform their functions; they need reassurance. In most cases initially adding technology will not result in a decrease of staff. Job duties and functions change and become more computer based.

With the introduction of change management and the efficiencies technology can add to your organization, you'll begin to assess how you can realize the benefits of the new technology. A technology training plan for clinical and administrative staff along with continual process redesign by an interdisciplinary, interdepartmental team bring improvements to daily operations. For example, nursing staff skilled in computer applications can more readily adopt the use of a computer network and a file management tool to access transcribed notes. An electronic access point to dictated reports and lab results reduces the need to pull physical records and eliminates delays for patients, both resulting in lower overhead costs and improved service. Another example of effective technology training and disbursement is the decentralization of appointment scheduling. Technology-trained nurses can schedule follow-up appointments for patients at the point of care rather than pushing the task to a check-out function where the authority to work in appointments to a capacity calendar is lacking.

Change in processes can be incorporated into the EHR training plan. Developing a training strategy involves answering three questions:

1. How will the training be conducted? Will the vendor, an internal trainer, or a combination of both teach the staff the re-engineered processes?
2. When will the training take place? Will you schedule training in phases or require employees to take one long training session?
3. How will the training be done? Will it be Web-based, conducted in small departmental groups, classroom style, on-site, or off-site?

Tips for successful training

Following is a list of tips to keep in mind when conducting staff training on a new EHR system or other new technology:

- Keep it simple — too many options on how to perform the same function may be overwhelming and confusing;
- Instruct trainers to be flexible and available and to provide a lot of one-on-one help (or smaller class sizes);
- Use real-life clinical and workflow scenarios in your training;
- Develop competencies surrounding implementation phases;
- Utilize super-users (staff members who are in-house experts) to assist users who may be having difficulties;
- Provide training assistance prior to go-live — hold "dress rehearsals";
- Develop a strategy for on-going training for new employees and those who need refreshers or who are having issues;
- Do not allow too much time before training and go-live without refreshers or assistance;
- Develop a training strategy and materials that encompass various competency levels (beginner, intermediary, advanced);
- Don't assume that a one-time, in-class session is sufficient for the go-live;
- Collect training feedback throughout the training program and incorporate it into the go-live planning; and
- Make sure that you have enough system content built and tested so that you can have a successful training program.

Departments and physical sites require a super-user. Clinical applications users will resort to prior methods if immediate help is not available. Don't expect staff to make a phone call to a help desk when an issue disrupts a patient encounter. Each location of clinical users will need a super-user as a go-to person to sustain the transition to the new technology. The use of technology is iterative in nature and the presence of a super-user will support that iterative effect. These super-users are vital to the system's implementation; they are an invaluable resource for the physicians and other employees and maintain the forward momentum of change required for the EHR adoption.

> ***Question:*** *"How do you eat an elephant?"*
>
> ***Answer:*** *"One bite at a time."*

The answer to this old adage is going to drive the change management plan for your EHR implementation. You will also benefit by taking advice from Stephen R. Covey's book, *The Seven Habits of Highly Effective People.*[1] Covey's second habit, "begin with the end in mind," will help as you begin thinking about implementation. "Begin with the end in mind" has to do with "purposes" but it also has a great deal to do with visualization and prior planning, which are necessary for complete planning. Any plan is better than no plan, but a plan poorly implemented can be financially and personally devastating.

Implementation failures

Implementing an EHR is a complex process that involves both cultural and organizational changes. In its report, *Extreme Chaos 2000*, the Standish Group reported system implementation projects, in general, experience low success rates.[2] They found that:

- 28 percent of projects meet full success;
- 49 percent of projects are fully completed, but are over budget, over schedule, and lack full scope of planned functionality; and
- 23 percent of projects experience complete failure or are cancelled.

Many change initiatives fail largely because employees feel left out of the process and end up lacking the motivation, skills, and knowledge to adopt new systems and procedures. The reasons are not usually technical; employees who are accustomed to the old ways of doing things reject the new. It is imperative that physicians enter the implementation stage prepared and ready to use the new technology. If the physicians will not use the technology or speak negatively about the changes, it is going to be extremely challenging for the staff to embrace it. The devil, as always, is in the details: how to implement change within your organization that takes human behavior into consideration.

There are various reasons for failure, some of the most common include:

- Lack of planning;
- Lack of executive support and commitment;
- Lack of resources dedicated to the project (for example, staff, time, money, end-user involvement, project management, and IT support);

Project Management Process Steps

1. Identify project team employees.
   a. Define roles.
   b. Communicate and prepare the practice.
2. Establish the EHR project goals.
   a. Establish strategies and scope.
3. Set project milestones and a realistic timeline.
   a. Identify activities and tasks.
   b. Estimate time and costs.
4. Deliver a quality product.

- Unrealistic expectations for what can be accomplished and how quickly it can occur;
- Relying on the vendor to assume responsibility for implementation;
- Expecting the new technology will fix operational and personnel problems; and
- A fear of change.

An EHR implementation is a major project; the management team must determine what needs to be done, how to accomplish these actions, do the work, measure the results, and bring the project to a close. The stakes are high and communication and planning are essential. Implementing an EHR will improve the quality of care and the efficiency of operations while decreasing costs. An example of an unsuccessful plan includes a do-it-in-your-spare-time mentality, lack of a dedicated project manager, and insufficient preparation.

Team members

A project or implementation manager needs to be identified. Ideally this person is someone with experience in planning who is also a good leader. This person must also be able to quickly adjust to changing conditions while remaining calm and focused. It is not a good idea to trust the project to an inexperienced but promising employee or an established manager with a full workload. A good project manager will take time to design necessary configurations and support and prepare providers and staff through this change process. Additional IDS implementation team members should include physician champions, departmental representatives (such as front and back office, clinical, diagnostic, and health information personnel), IT support, and trainers.

Ask the vendor to select and identify their project manager for your project. The vendor project manager is very important and should be identified early in the project planning. Each practice implementing the EHR will need its own project team with similar cross-departmental membership. The practice EHR team follows the guidance of the IDS project team while fulfilling all site responsibilities for implementation. The project plan needs to specify the responsibilities of the IDS project team and those of the practice site team.

Communication

Usually people are willing to change if they understand and accept the reasons, and have input into the way their jobs and workflow are restructured. Communication is one of the toughest issues in medical practices and integrated systems. Effective communication requires "shared meaning." Develop a written communication plan to ensure that all of the following occur within your change management process:

- Communicate consistently, frequently, and through multiple channels, including speaking, written memorandums, training, and your Intranet;
- Communicate all that is known about the changes, as quickly as the information is available;
- Encourage employees to ask questions, request clarification, and provide input;
- Clearly communicate the vision and the objectives of the EHR change management effort and help employees understand how these changes will affect them personally (if you do not clarify the changes, your internal grapevine will help with this process and spread misinformation, usually more negative than the truth);
- Recognize that true communication is a "conversation" (a two-way discussion must result); and
- Provide answers to questions only if you know the answer (it is much better to say you don't know, and that you will try to find out).

Start with defining requirements by documenting the processes (flow charts) within practices and across the IDS and obtaining feedback from key physicians and employees. The project manager should work with the staff to identify features that are "must haves" and those that are lower priority items. As mentioned earlier in this chapter, consider setting short (< 6 months), medium (6 to 12 months), and long (> 12 months) term goals, with measurable targets to help assess your progress toward those goals. Goals need to be realistic, attainable, and communicated to all, as well as take into account the current and future infrastructure of your practice. Are your goals focused on finance, growth, people, or customer service? Determine what efficiencies can be implemented to enhance processes.

Implementation strategy and scope

To determine the implementation strategy and scope of the implementation, each IDS needs to strategically address the following questions as one entity and also individually with each practice tactically, to determine alliances and necessary variances in the implementation:

- Do you want to utilize electronic charge capture, e-prescribing, or start with a chartless office?
- Is access from all office locations, hospital, and home crucial?
- Do you want to check billing codes to reduce rejected claims, reduce or eliminate transcription fees, improve patient safety and patient communication, or enhance workflow management?

- Is patient e-mail or Web access to the practice important?
- Do lab reports take forever to get into a patient's chart?

When determining your implementation strategy and scope you need to decide if you are going to incrementally phase in your use of the EHR or do a full-system implementation. Ambulatory EHRs are seldom successfully implemented in a "big bang" fashion. Most integrated systems utilize a phasing-in approach based on functionality, providers, related entities, or facilities/workflow implementation. Implement products/modules in a way that enables users to recognize incremental victories and obtain functionality in shorter time frames.

The transition to a chart-less office is a change that often is difficult to envision. Each entity must also address a medical records conversion strategy. What records need to be moved to the EHR system? How much historical information should be converted? Who will scan the charts and when? The physicians must decide if abstracting and manually entering certain patient data are needed. Successful change occurs when the paper chart conversion is completed by people with clinical experience and is validated prior to go-live by those who are familiar with patients' clinical history and treatments.

Paper chart conversion

The chart conversion period can last a full year past the EHR go-live week. Converting paper charts is a costly process. What are the options? Data, or information, can be stored in the EHR in two basic formats: discrete data or image data. It is important to understand the difference between these types of data and how it will affect future ability to access the information in the EHR.

Discrete data

Discrete data refers to individual pieces of information that are entered into specific fields in the EHR. Each piece of information has a unique place in the database. Every time this piece of information is entered into the EHR, it can be accessed in the EHR and can be reported upon.

For example, if the patient's weight is entered into the individual field for "patient weight" in the EHR, each weight at each visit can be compared to the last and displayed as a graph, list, table, etc. A patient has labs drawn at the hospital, and the report comes back with three results: INR 2.7, Potassium 4.0, and HbA1C 8.0. If these results are entered into the EHR as discrete data, the user will be able to view the lab results of today, compare them with the results from one month and two months ago, and graph them. It is important therefore to carefully consider what information should be entered discretely into the EHR.

As a general guideline, include as discrete data those pieces of information that will need to be easily accessed and compared over several patient visits. In addition, enter discrete data for information that will be used for report generation. Some examples of reports to run on a regular basis may include patients who are late for their yearly physicals, patients who need follow-up for high blood pressure, or performance measures of physicians for insurance companies.

Image or scanned data

Scanned data is information entered into the EHR as a block of text or an image (picture). It is filed in the EHR as a scanned document. Information entered into the computer by this method can be viewed and appears just as it did when it was scanned. The information cannot be compared or graphed by the EHR, as it is a picture of the information only.

For example, the patient's last physical exam document is scanned into the EHR. Within the EHR, the practice will be able to view the document to see what the patient weighed at that visit, but it will not be information that can be used in the EHR to compare against future weights entered during other patient visits. If that patient's lab results return with three tests and the results are scanned into the EHR, the practice can view that scanned report, but will not be able to compare or graph the test information, as it is only a picture of the page of lab results.

It is important to carefully consider what information should be entered into the EHR as scanned or image data. As a general guideline, only scan the historical information that will need to be referred to in order to care for the patient. Some examples of information to scan would be recent consult reports, a baseline and immediate past EKG reports, medical histories, discharge summaries, and correspondence from outside providers.

Use of a pre-load abstraction worksheet

Use of a standardized worksheet, such as the one shown in Exhibit 10.4, to extract clinical data from the record prior to the pre-load process can substantially speed up the actual entry of data into the EHR. When a pre-load worksheet is used, it is usually placed in the front of the chart so that the provider or a nurse can add the needed data to the worksheet as patients are seen in the office. This process can start as soon as the practice begins the implementation process. This can give the clinic up to three months to capture data on the patients. The data entry staff can then use the pre-load worksheets to enter data into the EHR rather than having to look through the record for the details and then add the information to the EHR. In addition, the practice can identify specific patients for which to complete the pre-load worksheet, independent of whether they are being seen for routine care during the pre-load period.

Once the vendor converts existing data from the old system into the new system, testing must be completed. You can *never* be too diligent when testing converted data. System testing is important, and conducting the following tests should be considered:

- Unit test (testing each component by itself);
- Integrated test (walking through your complete workflows including all interfaces);
- Stress test (testing the system at the capacity that you predict for normal daily use); and

EXHIBIT 10.4 ■ Sample Template to Organize Paper Record in Preparation of Pre-load

Patient Name: ______________________ **DOB:** ______________

Problem/Dx List

Description	Onset Date
Ex: Hypercholesterolemia	2003

Immunizations

Expand as needed to include other immunizations

Immunization	Date Given
Tetanus	
Pneumovax	
Hep B	
Meningitis	
Influenza	
MMR	
Polio	

Flowsheet

Description	Value	Date
Height		
Weight		
Blood pressure		
Cholesterol		
HDL		
LDL		
Trigylceride		
Pap smear		
Mammogram		
Bone density		
HgBA1c		
Sigmoidoscopy		
Colonoscopy		
Hemoccult		

(Exhibit continues on next page)

EXHIBIT 10.4 ■ Sample Template to Organize Paper Record in Preparation of Pre-load *(continued)*

Medication List

Description/Dose	Sig	Start Date
Ex: Lipitor 20mg	1 po qd	5/5/2005

Allergies

Description	Onset Date	Reaction
Ex: Penicillin	1995	Hives

Histories

Past Medical Hx:
Surgical Hx:
Family Medical Hx:

Social Hx:

Marital Status: Single		Married	Divorced Widowed
Children:			
Employment Status:			
Tobacco Use: Y	N	Previous Amount ___________	
Alcohol Use: Y	N	Previous Amount ___________	

- Parallel test (validating data against manual operations, such as paper medical records and encounter forms).

THE INTERNET IN MEDICINE

Manhattan Research performed a survey in January 2007 called "Taking the Pulse: U.S. — Physicians and Emerging Information Technologies."[3] The responses from 1,353 U.S. physicians demonstrated that 93 percent of physicians are using the Internet daily, and approximately 25 percent of physicians are accessing the Internet during patient consultations. Research also indicates that patients are becoming increasingly empowered as they gain more access to health information.

Medical practice executives often ask how they can use information management technology to help their organizations become an informatics leader. Clinicians often seek the technology that can help them learn about their patients. IT managers often question how clinical and non-clinical information relate within their organization.

The Internet provides all health care organizations with the opportunity to communicate with current and potential patients. Utilizing the Internet can improve practice efficiency and, more important, strengthen the physician–patient relationship. Each medical practice is unique; take time to discuss and design your Internet approach, and make certain it is centered on the needs of your IDS's practices and patients.

What are the differences between a Web portal and a Website?

A *Web portal* provides physician practices with an immediate presence on the Internet and a platform for integrating patients, practice partners such as health plans and hospitals, and vendors to your practices. A Web portal offers functionality such as marketing, interactive patient education, e-visits, and business process applications such as bill paying and e-billing statements. It also allows automated applications for lab and test results.

A *Website* is more static. Basically a Website may be seen as a marketing tool that is non-interactive and does not automate core business processes. Web portals on the other hand enable patients to securely contact their physicians or physician delegates and request medication refills and appointments. When linked to an EHR, patients can view or download certain components of their medical record (such as test results, medication, and problem lists). In addition, Web portals offer convenient asynchronous communication for both the patient and physician.

Take the time to aggressively educate your patient population about your Web portal. Put your Web address on statements, appointment cards, and brochures, and in your *Yellow Pages* advertisement. Instruct practices to change their on-hold messages to prompt patients to go online and/or use automated telephone tools. These tools (such as those for appointment reminders and lab result calls) can call patients to announce new features on the Website. You should also consider sending a "welcome" e-mail message to new patients that outlines the services offered on your Website. Many practices report that they have seen a reduction in physician phone traffic and a corresponding increase in practice efficiency.

A successful self-service technology strategy can strengthen every step of the patient care process at each of the IDS's practice sites. It is a natural next step to bring patient self-service to the check-in process. The numerous flaws of traditional paper-based methods are embarrassingly apparent. Patient misidentification and errors resulting from the duplicate manual entry of patient data, as well as poor service to our customers when we repeatedly ask for the same information can be avoided.

An automated patient registration process uses the swipe of a driver's license, credit card, or membership card to authenticate the patient's identity. Health Insurance Portability and Accountability Act (HIPAA) rules also require a second level of authentication, so patients can enter their Social Security number or birth date into the self-service device.

Some practices have added a biometric solution such as fingerprint imaging. Once patients are identified, they can begin checking in for the scheduled visit or lab test. They will then be required to enter or verify demographic, insurance, and medical history information. Patients can also pay their co-payments and past-due balances at the kiosk. This automation allows more dedicated staff time at both the IDS central office and at the practice sites to deal with patient questions and concerns, or for the performance of other productive activities. Several forms of self-service registration technologies are available, including wireless tablet computers, desktops, and freestanding kiosks. Many EHR vendors offer a supplemental portal product that can be delivered via kiosk as well.

CONCLUSION

The reality is that technology implementation does not end. Oversight and communication are two essential ongoing components of implementation. Consider keeping the EHR implementation team together but changing the focus. The team should continue to meet monthly and monitor quality issues. Ongoing issues include:

- Training (What training is available for new employees and providers? What training is available for system upgrades and process revisions?);
- Vendor's Web portal (Is there a portal? What services are offered?);
- User group meeting (Does the vendor offer an annual meeting?); and
- Online user support group (Does one exist? If yes, how do physicians and staff join? How does can the organization best utilize this resource?).

The focus on EHRs comes from a desire to reduce administrative costs and to improve services and quality of care to patients — do no harm. Frustration with the inadequacies of a paper-chart filing system drives providers in all delivery venues toward technology at an increasing rate.

The administrative burden in medical practices can be eased with the implementation of technologies to facilitate communication (for example, the provider administrative cost incurred per lab test is estimated at $19.25).[4] The practice of medicine is a business of communications. Communications can be facilitated by technology. Health care providers organized in medical practices, hospitals, and nursing homes have tremendous needs to effectively communicate within their organizations and between their organizations.

Implementation barriers to technology adoption in medical practices can be overcome by incremental approaches and knowledge transfer assistance from affiliated community health care partners, such as an IDS.

REFERENCES

1. S. Covey, *The Seven Habits of Highly Effective People* (New York: Free Press, 1989).

2. Standish Group International, *Extreme Chaos 2000* (Boston: The Standish Group, 2000).

3. Manhattan Research, "Taking the Pulse®: U.S. — Physicians and Emerging Information Technologies" (January 2007) www.manhattanresearch.com.

4. J. Walker, et al., "The Value of Health Care Information Exchange and Interoperability," *Health Affairs* (January 19, 2005).

CHAPTER ELEVEN

Management Selection

Richard D. Hansen, MS

Managing a medical practice requires a unique set of skills. While hospital administrators may have deep knowledge of inpatient operations, many struggle to successfully operate an ambulatory care organization. A medical group practice owned by an integrated delivery system (IDS) may have employed physicians and receive many administrative services from the IDS, but it is primarily a physician-based ambulatory operation. Physician practices, whether independent or owned by an IDS, require non-physician managers who work well with physicians but also convey the authority to supervise the nonclinical aspects of their practices. Although physicians are ideally suited to champion IDS goals and action plans at the ambulatory care level, very often the catalyst and the "glue" in that process is an effective administrator.

Finding the right practice administrator can be a time-consuming process. Because administrators leave employment for many reasons (such as retirement, advancement, or dismissal), it is critical to establish a succession and selection process that can identify the right person for the job.

In this chapter we discuss six steps to launching a successful search for the right administrator for the IDS–owned medical practice. These steps are:

1. Define the key roles of the practice;
2. List the key attributes of the ideal administrator/manager;
3. Define the compensation and benefits;
4. Plan to hire an interim administrator;
5. Define the recruitment protocol; and
6. Bring the new person on board.

We also discuss a strategy — hiring an interim administrator — to enable IDS leaders the breathing room in which to conduct an adequate search without disrupting the practice or practices the administrative position supervises.

STEP 1: DEFINE THE KEY ROLES OF THE PRACTICE

Before selecting an administrator or even defining the administrator's roles, it is important to define what he or she will lead. This definition can be found by asking the following questions:

- What are the goals of this practice or department and how do they support the IDS's overall vision, mission, and values?
- Are there specific components of the IDS's overall mission and purpose that this practice is — or can be — in the position to help fulfill?

Look to the business and marketing goals that have been established for this particular unit of the IDS to identify which portions of the IDS mission or business plan the practice is supporting.

Defining the practice's role in supporting the IDS also applies to other ambulatory units in which an administrator will supervise operations and providers (for example, an ambulatory surgery center, a physical therapy center, etc.).

Assess the medical practice

Each medical group has its own unique characteristics. These can be defined through three exercises:

- Conduct a brief SWOT (strengths, weaknesses, opportunities, and threats) analysis;
- List the practice's key priorities and challenges; and
- Identify where the practice's needs will draw upon the four general competencies of administrators identified by the American College of Medical Practice Executives (ACMPE) as necessary for competent performance in medical practice management.

The brief SWOT analysis may already have been performed for the IDS as part of a strategic planning exercise. That list can be amended as needed for each of its medical groups.

Describing in writing the organization's or medical group's key priorities and challenges (through the brief SWOT analysis) will give the recruiting committee or human resources staff a better idea of the qualities to seek in an administrator. Also it will inform candidates as to what they will be facing. In drawing up this list, it is important not to become overly focused on urgent short-term priorities to the exclusion of other important items, such as skills in financial management or operations. If the short-term needs are especially compelling (for example, the practice must rapidly expand into a new market), consider the option of hiring an interim administrator with deep experience in the priority area. Then, once the urgent short-term goal is moving forward, look for a permanent administrator to be the steady hand running the operation.

The four general competencies for success in medical practice management include:

- Professionalism;
- Leadership;
- Communication skills; and
- Critical thinking skills.

The administrative candidate search will benefit from knowing which of those competencies are needed most for the position. One medical group might be described as competitively aggressive or known for its political savvy in its market. This group may draw upon the administrator's competencies in business operations. Another group might be implementing an electronic health record that significantly changes its daily operations. This group would most benefit from an administrator whose skill set included technology implementation. (See the section, "Core competencies," found later in this chapter for more background into how these competencies are essential to performing the several domains of professional knowledge for the medical practice administrator.)

If the practice is already established, the description of its challenges and priorities would likely indicate the need for a leader who has solid operational experience, and someone who has managed more than one practice long enough to gain the skills and experience learned from accomplishments as well as mistakes. Established practices may also benefit from an administrator with good financial management skills who will take a steady approach to running day-to-day operations.

If the practice is a start-up by the IDS, there are other skills and experiences to consider in the administrative candidate. A new practice may benefit from the leadership of an administrator who has a "start-up" personality — someone who can think fast on his or her feet. Starting a practice requires creative thinking combined with persuasive skills. Physicians will need a leader who can help them adapt to changes in operations and technologies. Many start-up initiatives provide a testing ground for existing and potential physician leaders who can work jointly with the administrator to create an ideal practice environment.

If the practice is a recent acquisition, list the key areas where the IDS's strategic plan would likely lead to change in the medical practice. Knowing whether changes need to take place in the management structure, governance, performance, patient flow processes, or other areas can help create a realistic job description so that a candidate with the requisite experience is selected. The goals for the practice may already have been developed in strategic planning. Or, you may want the new administrator to help lead the way to a new strategic plan or business plan for the practice. The description of these goals can be specific (for example, "we want the practice to double in size to help the IDS attract more patients from this part of town") or it may be general (for example, "we want this practice to support our referral network"). This information will be helpful to administrative candidates and will also help IDS leaders to develop their interview process.

Prepare the candidate

Some of the documents developed during the practice assessment process are worth sharing with candidates. These documents may include:

- The foundational values and a brief mission statement of the IDS;
- The goals of the practice and its fit in the mission of the IDS;
- The IDS's organizational, governance, and leadership structure;
- The challenges and priorities of the practice; and
- The practice's business plan and pro forma.

This information can help potential administrative candidates get a more accurate snapshot of the challenges they may encounter on the job.

STEP 2: LIST KEY ATTRIBUTES OF THE IDEAL ADMINISTRATOR/MANAGER

Two important documents will emerge from the exercise of defining the practice's characteristics and fit within the IDS completed in Step 1:

- The administrator's job description; and
- The list of desired administrator qualities.

These documents will be critical to keeping the recruiting committee focused on finding the most suitable candidate for the position.

Before beginning a search for a new administrator, it is a good idea to survey the physicians — or the physician leaders in a larger practice — to determine what they expect from the individual who will be their administrator. Next, it is important to make sure these expectations are within the mission and goals of the IDS. The IDS's administrator in charge of physician practices, the organization's CEO, and other key leaders in the system should agree on the position's expectations. At this point it may be necessary to sit down with physician leaders in the practice to understand any differences they may have among either themselves or with the IDS regarding how the practice fits into the larger organization's vision. A lack of physician buy-in to or understanding of the IDS mission at this point may produce unrealistic expectations of the administrator and may lead to physician disenchantment later on.

A written job description helps to confirm the duties and responsibilities of the administrative position. When a long-time administrator leaves, this is the opportunity to review the position's responsibilities and duties and refocus them if necessary to better align them with the practice's current needs.

Core competencies

One of the most important contributions to the profession of medical practice management in the last decade has been the research conducted by the ACMPE that led to the development of the Body of Knowledge for Medical Practice Management. The ACMPE is the certification and professional development arm of the Medical Group Management Association (MGMA). By developing the Body of Knowledge for Medical Practice Management in conjunction with an expert panel of medical practice executives and input from hundreds of group practice managers, the ACMPE has defined and documented the professional competencies and areas of responsibility, or domains, required for successful medical group management. The competencies — professionalism, leadership, communication skills, and critical thinking skills — are themes that run throughout the profession's body of knowledge. (See Exhibit 11.1, "ACMPE Body of Knowledge Competencies Up Close" for information about the specific criteria in each skill set.) This body of knowledge is organized into major areas of responsibility. Currently there are eight defined domains:

- Business operations;
- Financial management;
- Human resource management;
- Information management;
- Organizational governance;
- Patient care systems;
- Quality management; and
- Risk management.

To varying levels a job may emphasize some or all of these domains of knowledge; however, the competencies of professionalism, leadership, and communication and critical thinking skills are a constant theme running through all of these domains. Many organizations find that the domains and competencies defined by the ACMPE are useful criteria for evaluating current administrators as well as potential administrators.

Beyond the basic competencies required for success in the position, it is also helpful to prepare a list of the specific qualities you seek in administrator (for example, decisiveness, ability to cope with multiple urgent demands, sense of humor etc.). The IDS management and the physicians in the practice should develop a single list of qualities that each party buys into. Listing those qualities makes it easier to evaluate candidates and can also double as an additional reality check to validate whether or not the physicians and the IDS are in alignment about the important goals and objectives for the practice.

Exhibit 11.2 illustrates an example of a chart to use in comparing and contrasting the IDS and practice's objectives with the desired qualities of a potential administrator.

The right "fit"

Finding the right administrator for an IDS– or hospital-owned practice is different than finding one for a private practice. A savvy and experienced administrator understands that a practice that is part of a large health system has different risks and rewards than a private medical practice. The entrepreneurial

EXHIBIT 11.1 ■ ACMPE Body of Knowledge Competencies Up Close

Professionalism: A commitment to achieving professional standards that enhance personal and organizational integrity and contribute to the profession. These skills include:

- Commitment to competence, integrity, altruism, and promotion of the public good;
- Commitment to self-assessment and continuous learning;
- Support for collegial relationships with peers through networking, information–sharing, and mentoring;
- Participation in and encouragement of service and volunteer activities to support the development of colleagues, staff, and the community;
- Demonstration and promotion of cultural sensitivity; and
- Demonstration of knowledge of the health care system and the environment in which it operates.

Leadership: Collaborating with and supporting the practice's physician leadership to provide strategic direction to the organization. These skills include:

- Upholding and advocating ethical standards and decision making;
- Fostering teamwork between clinical and administrative staff;
- Understanding effective techniques for working with boards and governance structures;
- Focusing on the implementation of organizational strategy;
- Inspiring others toward a shared vision;
- Supporting innovation and creativity;
- Demonstrating effective change management skills to ensure effective patient care and safety, as well as improving practice performance; and
- Understanding and effectively managing expectations.

Communication skills: Skills necessary to elicit multiple points of view from internal and external sources, facilitate constructive interaction, and present information clearly and concisely. These skills include:

- Writing clearly and effectively;
- Speaking clearly and effectively before individuals and groups in formal and informal settings;
- Developing effective interpersonal skills;
- Seeking out and incorporating the views of stakeholders for decisions that affect the quality of care, work environment, and business stability of the organization;
- Listening and responding effectively to the ideas and thoughts of others;
- Recognizing and using non-verbal forms of communication;
- Demonstrating effective negotiation and facilitation skills;
- Supporting and promoting effective conflict resolution; and
- Providing effective communication linkages within the organization and to its external environment.

EXHIBIT 11.1 ■ ACMPE Body of Knowledge Competencies Up Close *(continued)*

Critical thinking skills: A systematic, logical approach to problem solving, decision making, and the development and administration of systems to address day-to-day issues and the long-term improvement needs of the practice. These skills include:

- Collecting and analyzing data from internal and external sources relevant to each situation;
- Demonstrating the ability to discriminate between important and superfluous aspects of situations to support sound decision making;
- Asking the right questions when making decisions;
- Understanding cause-and-effect relationships;
- Learning from mistakes;
- Managing the overload of information and stress generated from diverse situations that occur in the practice and in your personal life; and
- Implementing planning methods and tools, including project management, process improvement, and systems thinking.

Source: Body of Knowledge for Medical Practice Management, Second Edition. Reprinted with permission from the American College of Medical Practice Executives (ACMPE), 104 Inverness Terrace East, Englewood, Colorado 80112. 877.ASK.MGMA. www.mgma.com. Copyright 2008.

spirit needed to succeed in private practice can translate well to a larger system, but some administrators from private practices struggle with the less-autonomous approach to decision making in a large system. Independent medical practices can be quite nimble in responding to the business environment because administrators are able to work closely with the physician leaders who own the practice. The relationship with top decision makers is much less direct in a large health system. A larger system, in other words, may frustrate some administrators. Experience in a large multispecialty group can provide a good background for success in a large IDS.

The business situation and local market will determine what other skills IDS leaders might place on their "must have" list of qualities for a practice administrator. For example, in an IDS comprised of numerous medical and surgical specialties, the skills and experience of managing a multispecialty group might be critical to the success of the practice. For an IDS that maintains medical practices in rural areas, a key factor might be how well the administrator fits into the community.

With a description of the practice and its needs (Step 1) and another list describing the desired skills and experience for the position (Step 2), the IDS is in a better position to determine which of the potential candidates are the right "fit." After that, the final decision often comes with a gut feeling backed by valid references.

EXHIBIT 11.2 ■ IDS Objectives and Administrator Desired Qualities

IDS Objectives	Administrator's Desired Qualities
Expand patient base to broader base of population in older urban areas	*Competencies* Collaboration *Skills* Marketing and planning Experience participating in service and volunteer activities Demonstrates performance in promoting cultural sensitivity
Bring physicians at recently integrated clinics into the system's culture	*Competencies* Leadership Communication *Skills* Effective interpersonal skills Able to inspire others toward a shared vision Able to manage change and assist others in coping with change
IDS–owned Practice Objectives	**Administrator's Desired Qualities**
Improve quality outcomes	*Competencies* Critical thinking Leadership *Skills* Fosters teamwork
Implement new electronic health record	*Competencies* Critical thinking *Skills* Previous success in project management

IDS — integrated delivery system

STEP 3: DEFINE COMPENSATION AND BENEFITS

Before initiating a search for a practice administrator, determine the pay range to offer to the individual selected. Most candidates have access to national surveys, including the annual MGMA *Management Compensation Survey.* They will expect to be paid accordingly based on their experience, the breadth of the job's responsibilities, and the size and complexity of the medical practice. If the position qualifies for bonuses, outline how they will be computed and awarded.

In many cases, the IDS will have a standard set of benefits for its personnel, including paid time off, pensions, insurance, and other benefits. An IDS may have all of its medical practice administrators in a standard pay plan that includes hospital and other management personnel. Some integrated systems set a job classification category for practice administrators to recognize that the position requires different skills and responsibilities than a hospital department administrative position. An additional reason to place practice administrators in a separate management category may be the opportunity to include bonuses based on the performance of the practice site or sites for which the administrator is responsible. Some sites may have substantially more complex operations than others and require a higher level of administrative skills. In either case, it is a good idea not to tie practice administrators' pay and benefits too closely to hospital positions because the duties and pressures are substantially different.

Plan on negotiating with candidates within a pay range that is based on the administrator's experience and other qualities, such as education, professional certifications, and achievements.

STEP 4: PLAN TO HIRE AN INTERIM ADMINISTRATOR

In almost all cases, the administrator of a medical practice — IDS–owned or not — is a major management function where selection should not be hasty. As such, IDS–owned medical practices may benefit in several ways from the use of a temporary administrator. When an administrator or other top-level executive leaves, an interim appointment can remove the pressure to find a quick replacement. While larger systems may have the capacity to assign this temporary responsibility to other managers, a medical practice requires intensive daily oversight. Hiring an interim manager can keep the practice on course while IDS leaders carefully recruit and vet candidates for the permanent position. An interim management position may well attract suitable candidates; namely, experienced medical practice administrators who find temporary assignments an opportunity for new challenges, change, and personal growth.

Temporary assignment terms

Administrators, information officers, financial officers, and other top-level managers working on a temporary basis can do more than babysit a practice; they can look at how management and other structures may need to change. They also can help create a game plan for the permanent administrator to follow.

Often, integrated systems find that bringing in an interim administrator can be an opportunity to review broader strategies. It can also be a chance to re-examine and possibly adjust the assigned responsibilities of the administrator position.

What's the ideal length of an interim administrative assignment? A term of five to eight months is not uncommon in an IDS–based engagement because it can take a while to get changes underway, such as reconfiguring staff ratios or implementing new processes. Also, the length of the interim term should be long enough to convince employees that they can't just ignore the temporary administrator. Longer assignments work well because employees in the practice will understand that they must work with and deal with the interim administrator; they will be less likely to form the attitude that they can put projects on hold until the permanent person comes on board.

Many IDS leaders find that an interim administrator can be an extra "pair of hands" to help implement a new project, as well as a "new pair of eyes" to spot ways to improve operations. An interim administrator who is from outside of the system may also provide a better perspective of what's going on in the practice.

It can take anywhere from a few days to a full month to locate an interim administrator. Management consultants who specialize in medical practice consulting may have connections with a broad base of experienced medical practice administrators. Finding qualified administrators who are willing to take interim assignments will require a nationwide search; a practice management consultant may be able to locate one in a matter of days or weeks.

IDS leaders can get additional value from an interim engagement by holding an exit interview with the interim administrator at the conclusion of his or her employment. A key question should be to list the top five issues that the permanent administrator will have to deal with during his or her first 12 months on the job.

What makes an interim administrator?

Flexibility and a willingness to try new things are certainly part of the makeup of an interim administrator. Other key attributes include:

- A proven track record;
- Excellent references;
- Long experience in medical practice management; and
- Willingness to seek new challenges.

As in hospitals, medical practices are continually facing challenging times. Mergers and acquisitions are among the reasons a qualified administrator may find him or herself suddenly in the job market. Some interim administrators are nearing retirement age but are still eager to work a few more years without having to relocate. Many just want new challenges and more variety; others view the temporary assignments as a chance to venture out in a new direction.

What to provide the interim administrator

In many interim arrangements, the temporary administrator is from out of town. The IDS should supply temporary housing, a meal allowance, and travel reimbursement for the individual to return home regularly — every other weekend is a common arrangement. Benefits, such as health insurance, retirement, vacation, and sick pay, are generally not part of these deals.

The salary depends on the administrator's experience. It may well be higher when computed on a monthly basis than a permanent administrator's combined wage and benefit package. Even so, the interim arrangement can be a good deal for the IDS because it brings in higher-level talent. More importantly, an interim arrangement allows the IDS to spend more time searching for the candidate who best matches the culture and management needs of the IDS, medical practices, or department.

The interim administrator's first 30 days

The first 30 days of the interim assignment is a critical time. The temporary position may require calming storms, implementing or recharging a stalled project, or even making important changes in the practice. Many IDS leaders find that interim administrators function well as change agents who can make hard decisions that a permanent manager may find difficult. Another role of the interim administrator is to lay the groundwork for the organization to reach a more stable state after hiring the permanent administrator.

Important details the interim administrator should be briefed about before his or her assignment begins are:

- To whom does he or she report?
- Who reports to the interim administrator?
- What are the primary duties and responsibilities of the engagement?
- How many days a week or month must the administrator be on site?
- What is the salary?
- Will travel and lodging expenses be reimbursed?
- Does the administrator have the authority to hire, fire, or reassign staff?
- What is the spending authority?

Once the arrangement is secured, a general timetable for the recruitment of the permanent person should be announced. This will make clear to everyone in the practice — physicians and staff — that a careful and extensive search has begun. IDS leaders can ease the uncertainties by announcing target dates for candidate selection and describing the framework of the search process.

The first order of business for the interim administrator should be to meet with the IDS executives who supervise the practice or department and with the top managers of the practice. Within days of arriving, the interim administrator also should meet with the key physicians and staff of the medical practices. The goal of these initial contacts should be to gauge the competencies of and gaps in the organization's staff.

Individual meetings with practice physicians, or at least with key physician leaders, can give the interim administrator a quick read of the practice's strengths, weaknesses, opportunities, and threats (also called a SWOT analysis). At this point, the information the IDS gathered in developing a portrait of the practice and its role within the IDS (discussed earlier in this chapter) could also be shared with the interim administrator.

At the beginning of the engagement, the top leader of the practice and the IDS liaison should list the outcomes they would like to see during the interim assignment. This can ensure that everyone has realistic expectations of what can and cannot be done in the short term.

Who's Qualified to be an Interim Administrator?

Unlike the person you select to fill a permanent position on your staff, there's almost no such thing as "overqualified" when it comes to an interim administrator. In fact, it might be wise to select an interim administrator who is clearly overqualified and has more experience than the person you will eventually hire.

Medical practices might be going through disruptive events such as changing strategy to align with the IDS's mission and goals, expanding or contracting in size, or implementing a new technology or process. When those situations occur during a change of administrative leadership, bringing in an overqualified interim administrator to manage the transition makes good sense.

An interim administrator with deep experience brings someone on board whom you might not be able to afford as a permanent hire. Plus, this person can come up with creative solutions, having already worked through similar issues and challenges at other jobs.

A highly qualified, even overqualified, interim administrator also will have:

- Credibility and smarts to deal effectively with physicians and employees concerned about recent management or ownership changes;
- Maturity to act as a peer to other managers; and
- The capacity to serve as a mentor to other managers and even to the person who eventually fills the administrative position.

An interim administrator can provide a high level of skill to a practice without getting in the way of (competing with) the organization's recruitment of a permanent administrator.

STEP 5: DEFINE THE RECRUITMENT PROTOCOL

The use of an interim administrator — whether recruited from outside or via an internal re-assignment — can give the IDS breathing room to develop the key components of the administrative leadership recruitment process, which include:

- A recruitment timetable,
- The recruitment committee, and
- A definition of the interview and selection process.

A reasonable timetable for recruitment may be anywhere from four to six months, but possibly longer. Creating a recruitment committee can help make sure that critical tasks are neither overlooked nor rushed. Consider appointing one or two physicians from the medical group or department, a member of the IDS executive staff that supervises ambulatory care practices, and perhaps a seasoned practice manager from one of the other groups owned by the IDS.

This committee can carry out recruitment tasks such as reviewing resumes, checking references, scheduling interviews, and recommending finalists to the IDS board of directors or whoever will make the hiring decision. A search firm can handle many of these steps; however, the entire process should not be handed over to outsiders. At least a portion of the tasks should be handled internally. It is important to find an individual whose personality, work style, and management approach meshes with the mission, vision, and values of the IDS as well as with the culture of the individual medical practice.

Advertise the position

Prepare an advertisement to announce the open position and its requirements. The first place to advertise is on the Website of the IDS. Locating administrators with the requisite skills to lead a medical practice, especially one that is part of a larger system, is frequently a national search. A management recruiter can help with the process by finding appropriate venues, including industry and professional Websites such as the MGMA Website, state MGMA Websites, local newspapers, and other forums. Management recruiters also will have their own networks of contacts but also should consult with the IDS to learn of additional contacts.

Qualified candidates may surface internally. If so, they should be considered along with outside candidates. While internal candidates bring a wealth of knowledge about the existing organization, outside candidates bring a new perspective. The qualifications of both need to be weighed to find the best fit for the IDS and the medical practice. No matter who is ultimately chosen, IDS leadership, physicians, and staff will be assured that they now have the best possible person for the job.

Select potential candidates

Within 30 days of the recruiting campaign, the recruitment committee should start meeting regularly to review resumes and draw up a list of potential candidates. A typical review process might follow the steps outlined in the following sections.

Conducting the initial review

The IDS's human resources department should be assigned to conduct a preliminary review of incoming resumes to screen out unqualified candidates. Allowing human resources professionals to assist also helps ensure that the search and review processes are conducted fairly to prevent the potential of an allegation of discrimination later on by an unsuccessful candidate.

The recruiting committee should then conduct the first review of qualified candidates' resumes by:

- Identifying potential candidates;
- Initiating brief screening interviews by telephone (either by conference call with the entire committee or by an assigned member of the committee with experience in interviewing);

- Selecting three to five top choices; and
- Checking at least three references for each candidate (including taking notes of references' comments).

The second review should consist of:

- Assessing references based on a compilation of comments received and the committee members' reactions;
- Narrowing choices to two or three candidates;
- Conducting a second round of telephone interviews; and
- Choosing two final candidates for on-site interviews.

Interviewing the candidates

The next important step is to conduct productive personal interviews with the top candidates. First, prepare an interview schedule for each candidate. Share the schedule with the practice's physicians, staff, and the candidate. Next, structure the candidate's visit. (Assign IDS staff as leads to oversee the details of each candidate's visit. These visits are paid for by the IDS.) Finally, schedule each recruitment committee member to conduct a one-hour interview with the candidate during the visit.

Although preparing the schedule and structuring the visits can be assigned to IDS management staff, the commitment to be available for and conduct the one-hour interviews should be part of the expectations for search committee members. If the committee has several members — more than eight — consider holding small group interviews to avoid a drawn-out interview process. It is not uncommon for applicants to top management positions like this to experience several hours of interviews over a one- or two-day period. Be careful not to schedule more than seven or eight interviews on any one day.

To ensure that the interview process leads to an informed selection decision, it is important to perform these additional activities:

- Schedule key management staff for 30-minute interviews with candidates (in some cases interviews may be in groups);
- Give the physician leaders in the medical group the opportunity to meet the candidate over lunch, dinner, or at another social gathering; and
- Arrange for the recruitment committee to host a candidate dinner for social interaction — you can learn a great deal about someone during such events.

As an obligation of serving on the recruitment committee, each member should be well-prepared to participate fully in the interview and assessment processes. This includes scheduling adequate time for these activities. It also includes knowing pertinent statistics about the medical practice or department, such as the number of patients seen per day, number of surgeries/deliveries/procedures per year, collection rate, and employee turnover rate. A capsule view of the practice, and the IDS's position in the marketplace, should be enough to help a professional administrator determine the financial health of the practice and the organization that owns it.

If you go to the expense of bringing in an administrative candidate for interviews, it's critical to leverage that expense by preparing an agenda that essentially scripts out the candidate's visit. Interview the candidate on a work day so that he or she can see the practice in operation. Allow time for the candidate to speak with all of the physician partners, when feasible, and the primary staff members (or at least those who will make the employment decision). A professional administrator will look just as hard at his or her potential work environment as you look at him or her.

Following up

Within 24 hours of the on-site interviews, schedule time for the committee members to provide feedback to each other and make a recommendation about the candidate's potential fit within the medical practice and the IDS. Be sure to inform candidates about the timeline for making the hiring decision.

As this process is repeated for each of the top candidates, a ranking order will start to emerge. Often, a favorite seems to rise head and shoulders above the other finalists. If you can choose a candidate at this point, contact the person as soon as possible about your decision. Don't procrastinate or you may lose the candidate — good administrators often have more than one practice interested in them. Follow up with a written offer that describes compensation, benefits, starting date, etc. Have a term sheet prepared that states the position's salary, the bonus (if any) and how it's calculated, and a summary of the benefits.

Allow up to 72 hours for a response. If the candidate accepts, inform everyone in the practice. If not, decide whether you want to hire the second candidate. If yes, proceed as with the first candidate. If not, go back to your short list and reconsider those individuals.

If the lead candidate is hired elsewhere or declines the offer, carefully consider the other candidates. If none seem right, continue the recruiting process. Be sure to inform those candidates invited for the in-person interviews that the hiring deadline has been extended. At this point, the recruitment committee may wish to consider whether to make changes in the hiring approach for this position. Is the compensation reasonable? Does the IDS, the medical practice, or department have internal issues that make candidates back off? Is the administrator position being given enough authority and latitude to attract the candidates the IDS most wants to hire?

STEP 6: BRING THE NEW PERSON ON BOARD

After the candidate accepts your offer, develop a plan for ongoing communication until he or she arrives at the practice. Assign one IDS executive staff person to oversee communication with the new administrator. Inform the incoming administrator of any key decisions made during the interim period.

Put out the welcome mat

Making the new administrator feel welcome in the practice and in the community is an important part of retaining that person. Just as the recruitment committee formed quick first impressions of the applicants, so, too, are impressions of the practice being formed on the administrator's first few days.

Schedule time for the new administrator to meet practice physicians and staff during the first week on the job. Schedule at least one welcome-to-the-community event that includes the new administrator's family. Work with the new administrator to schedule introductory meetings with key personnel in the medical practice and within the IDS as a whole. Find ways to introduce the new administrator to important outside stakeholders, such as managers at major referral sources not directly affiliated with the IDS. Often, local medical managers have professional networking associations; encourage the new administrator to join and participate.

Orientation

Structure regular orientation and feedback sessions with the new administrator during his or her first year. Designate a physician leader in the practice to meet with the new administrator at least once each week during his or her first two or three months on the job. Regular meetings with the physician or practice administrator at the IDS also should be scheduled. It is important that the administrator understand the broader operations of the IDS, so visits to key sites should be scheduled. Most integrated systems include practice administrators in regular management meetings.

Evaluations

Conduct formal evaluations to take place during the new administrator's first year at intervals of 3, 6, and 12 months. Also at these evaluations, touch base with the physician leaders in the medical practice to gain their input in evaluating the new administrator. These leaders can contribute to the assessment and confirm whether the administrator has achieved his or her goals. They also can provide qualitative input that can reflect on issues such as management style and demeanor.

CONCLUSION

While organizations may have their own approaches to recruiting administrators, it is important the IDS follow a process — one that is understood by the medical group and the candidates under consideration. It also is important for the IDS to modify its recruitment and interview process as needed to meet the unique needs of finding the best match for the medical practice or department. It may well be a different process than what is needed to find a hospital-based manager. In selecting an administrative leader for one of its owned medical practices, the IDS may need to include employed physicians as appropriate in the recruitment process and/or the administrator's performance evaluation process.

Recruiting the ideal administrator for an IDS–owned medical group practice requires a protocol that is at least somewhat different than that used to search for hospital administrators. Implementing a distinctive protocol helps ensure a successful outcome for the medical practice and the IDS.

CHAPTER TWELVE

Rural Delivery Systems

Trip Kinmon, FACMPE

Integrated delivery systems (IDS) in rural communities — the "new frontier" — continue to grow and develop in sophistication. Established initially on smaller scales, they are beginning to incorporate most of the sectors of the health care industry serving rural communities, including hospitals, physicians, medical groups, nursing homes/long-term care facilities, and even network payer agreements and relationships.

The development of rural integrated systems is a response to the unique challenges that hospitals, health care delivery systems, and physicians face in remaining economically viable sources of health care in their communities. The populations they serve are often in remote locations, with few resources to support an IDS's infrastructure. It is often necessary for these rural systems to recruit not only health care professionals, but also support staff as well. Other rural systems find themselves on the outer fringes of expanding metropolitan areas where they come into direct competition with large, well-established, well-funded urban-based systems.

The importance of hospital-based systems to rural communities is considerable. They are the anchors of these communities. Health care employment is often a stable contributor to the economic health of rural communities. Rural hospitals and rural health systems may be among the largest employers in the communities they serve and, therefore, have the potential to significantly affect economic stability as well as the overall health of those communities. The physicians who rely on these institutions also are important employers in rural areas. According to a study by the National Center for Rural Health Works, one physician employed in a rural community is estimated to add 23 jobs to that community. In the aggregate, these jobs pay out approximately $900,000 in salary and benefits and generate $1.5 million in revenue on average.[1]

As such, rural health systems are significant contributors to the economies of their communities. They may also represent the foundations of the education system, cultural interests and activities, and the pool for positions of civic and community leadership. This economic position gives rural health systems ample opportunity to leverage their unique and central community roles to successfully deal with the many economic and recruiting challenges these, typically smaller, systems face.

CHALLENGES FOR RURAL HEALTH CARE SERVICES

Providers and hospitals serving rural communities face a number of economic challenges. Rural communities have increasingly higher percentages of older residents compared with urban areas, as younger and higher educated people tend to move to where there are more jobs.[1] Because the elderly tend to consume health care services at a higher rate than younger populations, rural health systems must offer a broader base of services to accommodate that demand if they are to keep these services within their communities.

Many of those who are moving to rural communities are foreign-born and foreign-trained, which presents other issues to those communities such as cultural fit and language barriers.[2] These foreign-born individuals and their families are often drawn to available, low-skill jobs.

Rural areas also have a higher percentage of small business economies than urban areas. And as small businesses increasingly drop employee health coverage, the lower rates of employee-sponsored insurance contributes greatly to the lower rate of insurance for rural children and working adults.[3]

Rural hospitals and physicians are more likely to accept Medicare or Medicaid patients and, therefore, tend to have a higher proportion of these patients than urban physicians.

Recruiting physicians to rural areas

With the many existing and increasing demands for health services in rural communities comes the greater need for more and better trained health care professionals. Yet, graduating medical residents show a disinclination to seek out professional opportunities in rural areas. As the population ages in rural communities, so does the health care workforce. There is a risk that the health care workforce will begin retiring at about the same time demand for its services begins to increase. While the percentage of the population 65 and older in rural areas continues to rise, the percentage of those in the 18 to 30 age group is falling in many communities. This raises concerns about whether rural communities will be able to retain and train health care professionals and the support personnel they need.

A chief concern about rural provider shortages is the fact that primary care physicians and allied health care professionals are, along with the community hospital, foundations of the rural health care delivery system. They employ staff, pay benefits, and create collateral job opportunities for the community. These physicians also support the hospital in their community. The strength of the primary care base often can increase the need for specialty and subspecialty service availability in the community. As more specialty services are available in the community, a higher percentage of health care demand is served in that community.

When a physician shortage causes residents to seek health care services — specialty, ancillary, or primary — elsewhere, not only does the health care economy of the community suffer, so also does the economy in general because other purchases made while accessing health care out of town are also lost to the local community. This out-of-town shopping for health care can lead to established patterns of accessing care. Once these patterns are firmly established, it is very difficult to reverse them.

Many rural communities have come together to support their hospitals and health systems by assisting with capital development, physician recruitment, and, equally important, physician and allied health professional retention. Unlike larger communities, many rural hospitals tend to work more closely with their local businesses to find jobs for family members, introduce those families to schools and churches, and help with recruitment and retention issues. Rural communities often dedicate a higher percentage of their budgets to recruitment and retention than do hospitals in urban areas.

Among the attractions of a rural hospital, such as more independence and practice autonomy, physicians may have a greater ability to care for their patients. For example, in several rural communities in the United States, family medicine physicians are not only able to deliver babies, but also they are given C-section privileges at local hospitals. These privileges rarely exist for family medicine physicians in larger, urban communities.

A rural-based IDS can emphasize to potential physician recruits the lower-stress style of living and the higher purchasing power possible in rural areas. With the lower cost of living in rural areas, rural physicians have more purchasing power. One recent study found that the average income of rural physicians adjusted for the cost of living was significantly higher than that of urban physicians — $225,000 vs. $199,000, which translated to approximately 13 percent more purchasing power for the rural physician's income compared with the urban physician.[4]

Rural hospital development

Many hospitals in rural areas were established as quasi government, district hospitals. Communities assumed a role in establishing these hospitals. More recently, in the late 1990s, the federal government established provisions for Critical Access Hospitals (CAH), providing for cost-based reimbursement from Medicare, as opposed to Prospective Payment System reimbursement, which allows hospitals to recover capital costs in reimbursement. This enabled rural hospitals to more realistically provide much needed facilities and infrastructure in which physicians could practice and care for their patients — keeping them in the communities they served. Hospitals were able to shore up their financial positions and devote resources to recruiting physicians. The circle, or demand spiral, continued as hospitals and their medical staffs grew, providing health care for growing communities.

THE SMALL-SCALE RURAL DELIVERY SYSTEM

While difficulties recruiting and retaining physicians to rural areas continue, physicians and integrated systems have begun to work together, pooling talent and resources, in meeting the physician supply shortage in rural areas. This pooling of resources has evolved into a health care phenomenon — integrated systems on a small scale. The "small-scale" IDS is often more nimble and responsive to opportunities and, therefore, offers physicians more opportunities to meet their needs.

These small-scale integrated systems look in many ways like the larger, more sophisticated versions found in urban areas. Smaller integrated systems may have several advantages over the larger systems in terms of community support. Rural hospitals, CAHs, and integrated systems in rural areas report that they are more successful in recruiting and retaining physicians to their communities when the community's leaders, not just the health care leaders, are involved in the these efforts.

Smaller integrated systems, frequently in rural settings, are often not burdened with an oversupply of physicians and health care infrastructure. It may seem odd to refer to this "undersupply" as an advantage. It is, however, an oversupply of physicians and health care infrastructure that creates overhead, or costs, that must be spread throughout the system. The oversupply creates unnecessary competition, a dilution of the market potential for each provider or element of the system, and resulting dissatisfaction. At least in an undersupply environment, the system has the opportunity to grow to meet the demand. That growth keeps the IDS vibrant and the local economies healthy.

Smaller integrated systems are often not encumbered with the formality of process and the bureaucracy of protracted decision-making policies. Their boards are typically lay boards (comprised of members of the community) that are largely very supportive of the hospital's and the IDS's leadership. Members of these boards are physicians and business and community leaders, particularly in small, rural communities, and are accustomed to making decisions in their daily business lives. Physicians, who are decision makers by nature and training, often find working in an IDS environment with these nimble qualities more satisfying than do their counterparts working in larger, less nimble integrated systems.

EVOLUTION OF THE SMALL-SCALE RURAL DELIVERY SYSTEM

Many rural hospitals that evolved into integrated systems on a smaller scale did so in response to market conditions, particularly with regard to recruiting physicians. Frequently, physicians would find their practices struggling with the realities of a downturn in the local economy or competition from regional medical centers. Reimbursement also would become a challenge. Often inadequate staffing would cripple a physician's practice and his or her ability to meet the community's service demands.

These rural physicians, like their urban counterparts, look to the local hospitals for assistance. Options for partnerships include services under a management agreement for a management services organization (MSO), practice acquisition, or physician employment. Other options include assistance in establishing a freestanding rural health clinic (RHC) for the practice, if it is primary care in nature. If the practice becomes hospital-affiliated, or hospital-employed, options include establishing a provider-based RHC or a provider-based clinic.

Management services organization

MSO services might be the first phase of the relationship, or service model, defined as an IDS. Hospitals provide an array of management and operations support services through a formal management agreement to physicians for a fee. The goal of the MSO is to enhance physician–hospital relations by providing support without competition and interference. The provision of MSO services is often the first step a hospital takes in developing an IDS, and this progression is seen in many rural areas.

MSO agreements must meet regulatory requirements and tests, but they are essentially services provided for a fee. Hospitals began to provide these services to physicians because physicians lacked the capital, expertise, desire, or are otherwise unwilling or unable to effectively provide services for their practices.

As in urban areas, there is a steep learning curve as hospitals discover a distinct difference between the details of physician practice operations and hospital operations. If not effectively managed, MSO initiatives can represent financial losses for hospitals and hospital-owned systems. In addition to financial losses, poorly planned or executed MSO strategies run the risks of losing goodwill with physicians and, in some cases, of falling afoul of federal regulations.

Rural Health Clinic

The RHC program was established in 1977 to increase primary health care services to Medicare and Medicaid patients in rural communities. These clinics may be private, public, or not-for-profit. The primary advantage of the RHC program is increased reimbursement for providing Medicare and Medicaid services to rural areas. Increased reimbursement is intended to be the incentive to provide and expand primary care to target areas. The RHCs must be located in rural, underserved areas in order to qualify for the designation and they must incorporate the services of mid-level primary care practitioners.

A practice contemplating RHC status must be located in a rural area, which is an area not designated by the U.S. Census as an "urbanized area." The Rural Assistance Center (RAC) and the Centers for Medicare & Medicaid Services (CMS) provide resources to assist a practice in determining whether or not it meets the rural area test. The State Office of Rural Health found in states may also be a resource. The medical practice's state agency responsible for RHC certification and the CMS regional office provides final determination as to whether or not a practice passes the test.

The RHC must be located in a shortage area as so designated within the past three years. Three types of shortage areas qualify:

- Federally designated health professional shortage areas (HPSAs);
- Federally designated medically underserved areas (MUAs); and
- State governor-designated and secretary of Health and Human Services-certified areas.

Practices may ask for assistance from their state agencies responsible for RHC certification to determine status. They may research the Health Professional Shortage Area database, Medically Underserved Area database, and contact their state Office of Rural Health.

RHCs use a team approach to providing care to the patients served. The team includes physicians, nurse practitioners, physician assistants, and nurse midwives to provide care. The RHC must be staffed at least 50 percent of the time with mid-level practitioners. The RHC provides outpatient primary care services and basic laboratory service. The RHC may provide other services, but the reimbursement for those services may not be at the same rate as other RHC primary care services.

The increased reimbursement may result from special Medicare reimbursement based on the costs to provide services. The concept is that the volume of service, therefore access, provided is increased through the use of mid-level practitioners. Medicaid reimbursement may be increased, as it is based on the cost-based Prospective Payment System. Ordinarily this results in an increase in reimbursement. Again, the assumption is that volume will increase as a result of the utilization of mid-level practitioners. There is the assumption that their use will result in a more efficient clinic operation.

RHC certification may not always result in improved reimbursement. A detailed analysis of the services provided and the costs associated with providing those services is necessary. In some cases, traditional fee-for-service reimbursement is better. Much depends on the practice's payer mix. It is advisable to consider the services of a professional experienced in RHC matters in evaluating the financial feasibility of establishing one of these clinics.

Freestanding Rural Health Clinic

A freestanding RHC may be any primary care physician or group practice that meets the requirements of minimum number of primary care physician and mid-level practitioner providers and the rural test requirements mentioned in the previous section. These freestanding RHCs process their RHC claims payments through a fiscal intermediary (several of which are contracted through CMS throughout the country to provide these services) or a Medicare administrative contractor (MAC). The process for determining eligibility for RHC status is as described earlier in this chapter.

Provider-based Rural Health Clinic

Provider-based RHCs are clinics that are considered an integral part of a hospital, nursing home, or home health agency that is already a Medicare-certified provider. The provider, hospital, etc., handles reimbursement for the RHC. The requirements for receiving the designation are as described in the previous sections.

Provider-based clinics

Physicians electing employment with a hospital or IDS may find that their practice qualifies as a provider-based clinic. Employment by a hospital or IDS does not, in itself, qualify a physician practice as provider-based. The reward for following the processes for qualification, application, and attestation is increased Medicare reimbursement for the physician's professional component of services provided, and potentially for the hospital's facility component. Physician services provided in a traditional freestanding practice setting are billed and reimbursed through the Medicare Physician Fee Schedule.

In a designated provider-based setting, services are reimbursed in two parts:

- The hospital facility payment under the ambulatory payment classification (APC) rate for the outpatient hospital services; and
- A separate payment for the physician's services paid under the Medicare Physician Fee Schedule but reduced for the hospital site-of-service.

The result, the combination of the APC payment and the reduced Medicare Physician Fee Schedule payment, may be greater than the global professional fee reimbursement for the traditional freestanding clinic. This split payment requirement is viewed by many as a disadvantage of establishing a provider-based clinic because of the potential patient confusion it causes with Medicare patients. A further disadvantage is that this split payment methodology may require Medicare patients to pay two deductibles if they did not otherwise obtain hospital inpatient or outpatient services during a deductible period.

While the IDS offers the opportunity for provider-based clinic status, and the increased total reimbursement described earlier, not every practice may benefit. Certain specialties already practice in a provider-based setting (such as emergency physicians, pathologists, radiologists, and anesthesiologists) and are already subject to the provider-based billing and payment methodologies. Some specialty and sub-specialty services are reimbursed better under the traditional freestanding payment method than they are under the Medicare Part B and APC payment methodology. It is necessary to undergo a detailed service and payment analysis to determine whether or not provider-based status offers an advantage. If the advantage — increased reimbursement — is not significant, it may not be worth the effort and continued operational requirements to obtain provider-based status.

Some practices may not be eligible for provider-based status. The basic eligibility requirement is that the practice must be owned and operated by the hospital. Physicians and group practices that are completely independent do not qualify unless they dissolved, sold, restructured, and became employees of the hospital.

A provider-based clinic associated with a critical access hospital (CAH) receives reimbursement for its Medicare patients differently. Instead of receiving Medicare Physician Fee Schedule reimbursement and APC payments, the hospital (provider) receives the hospital's (provider's) Medicare Cost Report, and a physician payment under the physician Medicare Physician Fee Schedule, reduced by the hospital site-of-service. The resulting total payment may well be greater than the global reimbursement for the traditional freestanding setting, but the provider-based status addition to the CAH Medicare Cost Report could result in a negative impact. Some of the hospital's operating costs will be allocated to the provider-based clinic, while they were fully allocated to more costly hospital operations prior to provider-based status. A thorough analysis of costs and reimbursement must precede a determination to establish a provider-based clinic. Again, this analysis should be made by those experienced in such matters.

Disadvantages

While it appears that the advantages of the provider-based status are significant, there are disadvantages as well. The biggest disadvantage is the apparent loss of independence and autonomy that comes with employment. This is often a very bitter pill for physicians to swallow. Experience suggests, however, that the pill may not be as bitter in smaller, rural integrated systems as in larger, more urban systems. Physicians, hospitals, and integrated systems in rural settings tend to have closer, more aligned relationships than their more urban counterparts. Experience further suggests that relationships entered into for the right reasons are the healthiest relationships.

The greatest disadvantage to converting to provider-based billing status is "change." If the physicians are not already employed by the hospital, they must undergo a cultural change. For some physicians, this change is too great. For others, if the employment relationship with the hospital or IDS is done well, the change is not as difficult. Experience has proven that employment models can be developed to successfully address the fears physicians might have in "giving up autonomy" in exchange for hospital employment.

Another perceived disadvantage of establishing a provider-based clinic is that the provider-based clinic must be a department of the hospital. It must appear to patients, in no uncertain terms, that it is a department of the hospital. For physicians who were already employees of the hospital, this requirement may not be a problem. However, for physicians who were once independent, becoming employed by the hospital in order to obtain provider-based status can be a major hurdle. Establishing the relationship properly from the outset can minimize this obstacle.

Other requirements

There are other requirements for a practice to qualify as a provider-based clinic that physicians not accustomed to inpatient, or hospital, medicine may find difficult. These include:

- Compliance with Emergency Medical Treatment and Active Labor Act (EMTALA) requirements;
- Proper billing of physician services with the "site-of-service" indicator so that the Medicare site-of-service payment reduction can be properly applied;
- Compliance with all the terms of the hospital's and provider's Medicare provider agreement;
- Compliance with Medicare's non-discrimination provisions;
- Treatment of all Medicare patients as hospital outpatients for billing purposes;
- Subjecting billings for Medicare patients to the 72-hour payment window applicable to Prospective Payment System hospitals (this requirement does not apply to CAHs); and
- Compliance with Joint Commission standards and requirements where the hospital is so accredited.

Attestation process

The attestation process — the provider's attesting to certain operational matters associated with the proposed provider-based practice — is quite detailed and should be completed with diligence and care. The attestation statement identifies the hospital and provider, and makes it clear (through reference to services, patient flow, and identity) that the proposed provider-based clinic is, indeed, a department of the hospital. The hospital's bylaws and governing policies will apply to the provider-based clinic, and it must be demonstrated, through the attestation process, that there are no obstacles, or barriers, to this in obtaining provider-based status. The organization chart and job descriptions of all employees of the proposed provider-based clinic, including physicians, must demonstrate a connection to the provider's organizational and operational systems. Communication must be demonstrated to be uninterrupted and readily available to all departments of the provider at all times. The attestation process will provide evidence that the provider has communicated to the community and all patients served — in particular Medicare patients — that the provider-based clinic is a department of the hospital.

While formal approval of provider-based status is not required before billing as such, it is strongly recommended that the hospital, or IDS, considering such status follow the process of providing a detailed attestation statement to CMS and the hospital's regional administrator to obtain acknowledgment and approval before billing. This process ensures that if the system intends to "walk like a duck" (provider-based clinic), it "quacks like a duck" (to CMS' ears). While completing the detailed attestation process, a thorough financial analysis should also be performed to determine with relative certainty that there will be a financial gain with provider-based status sufficient to offset the disadvantages.

QUALITIES OF A SUCCESSFUL RURAL INTEGRATED DELIVERY SYSTEM

IDS strategies in rural communities can offer many advantages for the hospital and the physicians involved, but integration strategies also can create serious physician–hospital relationship challenges between physicians involved with the IDS and physicians in the private community who are not aligned, or involved, in the integration strategies. If we assume that the integrated strategy was well thought out and has the potential for positioning the IDS well in the IDS's service area, these challenges must, at the outset, be successfully dealt with.

One characteristic of an IDS with a successful medical staff relationship is effective communication. The period in which hospitals and physicians competed and developed strategies for unilateral advantage has, for the most part, passed. There is now more coordination and collaboration to accomplish mutually beneficial goals — health care for the communities they serve. When strategies evolve that appear to run counter to coordination and collaboration, it is essential that IDS leadership thoroughly commit to communicating the intent and benefit of the strategy. Failure to make this commitment could be catastrophic for physician–hospital relations with the independent physicians on staff. A reminder: those non-aligned physicians also serve the community. Communication is essential in every relationship, no matter how difficult or time consuming the task may be.

IDS administration in rural settings might not be experienced in all operational aspects of IDS models. Frequently these hospitals, and emerging systems, find themselves employing physicians for the first time. In order to develop the systems effectively, they often seek advice from colleagues, neighboring rural integrated systems, or consultants. One of the most important strategies for these systems is to partner with physicians in order to understand the complexities of medical group management.

Successful IDS administrators have the support of their boards and communities and are able to act quickly, effectively, and with support when they undertake new projects, or execute new strategies, that benefit the hospital, the system, and the community. If it is necessary to obtain advice or help in executing these strategies, these administrators and systems are typically nimble enough to make decisions and execute.

CONCLUSION

As health care continues to become more and more competitive in fully developed urban settings, the option of practicing in an IDS model in rural settings will become more and more attractive to physicians. As the primary care physician base becomes more fully developed within these rural integrated systems, specialists and sub-specialists will be recruited to the rural systems. These specialists and sub-specialists will fuel further growth of integrated systems to include ambulatory surgery centers, diagnostic imaging centers, and physician medical office building development.

REFERENCES

1. National Center for Rural Health Works, "The Economic Impact of a Rural Primary Care Physician and the Potential Health Dollars Lost to Out-Migrating Health Care Services," National Center for Rural Health Works, www.ruralhealthworks.org (accessed Sept. 12, 2008).

2. A. Kirschner, E.H. Berry, and N. Glasgow, "The Changing Demographic Profile of Rural Areas," *Rural New York Minute* (January 2009), http://devsoc.cals.cornell.edu/cals/devsoc/outreach/cardi/publications/upload/01-2009-RNYM.pdf (accessed March 11, 2009).

3. Health Resources and Services Administration, "Why is Rural Important? Enrolling Rural Children in CHIP and Medicaid," The Rural Work Group of the Interagency Task Force on Children's Health Insurance Outreach (1999), http://ruralhealth.hrsa.gov/pub/chip2.htm (accessed March 11, 2009).

4. J.D. Reschovsky and A. Staiti, "Physician Incomes in Rural and Urban America," Center for Studying Health System Change (January 2005), www.medicuspartners.com/pdfs/Rural_vs_City_2-5_Article.pdf (accessed Dec. 1, 2008).

CHAPTER THIRTEEN

How to Market the Integrated Delivery System

Kenneth T. Hertz, CMPE

The concept of marketing in health care organizations gradually developed in the late 1970s. It came into its own in the 1980s. In its earliest incarnation, marketing was employed to increase patient flow and volume as more patients meant more revenue. Today, the marketing function in health care organizations is accepted as integral and appropriate, and while it continues to have importance in driving patient volume, it now is seen as critical to enabling the institution, whether large or small, to differentiate itself from other organizations.[1]

This chapter describes the process of marketing as it exists in health care today. Starting with the basics of marketing — positioning and branding — the chapter progresses through the components of strategic marketing and the development of a strategic marketing plan. This chapter also focuses on and explores the opportunities and challenges inherent in the development of a marketing initiative within an integrated delivery system (IDS).

While we often use the term "customer" and mean "patient," we must also understand that in an IDS, our customers are varied. *Customers* may be patients, employers, insurers, or other physicians. Throughout this chapter we use the term "customer" in the broadest sense of the word unless otherwise noted.

WHAT IS MARKETING?

The American Marketing Association defines marketing as "the activity, set of institutions, and processes for creating, communicating, delivering, and exchanging offerings that have value for customers, clients, partners, and society at large."[2] Marketing is not, as many people believe, advertising or public relations. Marketing is a process, a transaction in which at least two parties are involved. In the case of health care, these two parties might consist of a physician's office and a new patient, or an IDS and local employers.

In each of these examples there are two parties, offerings of value, and customers and clients. The physician office may employ marketing to bring new patients into the practice. Tactics employed include advertising in various media, local sponsorships of organizations or events, and public speaking engagements. The goal is to bring more patients into the practice, generate more services, and increase revenue. This is a typical model for marketing items such as automobiles and tennis rackets or services like restaurants and health care.

The previous example focuses on the institution and generating more "sales." The IDS may consider an alternative approach with employers. In this case, the emphasis is on the needs of the employer (the customer). This customer-centric approach seeks to position and "brand" the IDS on the service value of the institution. The American Marketing Association defines a *brand* as a name, term, sign, symbol, or design, or a combination of these. The intent of a brand is to identify and differentiate the goods or services of an organization from its competitors. In terms of marketing an IDS, we're not going after more individual office visits as much as we want to create a powerful picture for the customer, displaying the IDS's strengths in areas including quality of care, customer service, or ease of access. We seek to position the IDS in the mind of the consumer as Brand Number 1.

In their groundbreaking book, *Positioning: The Battle for Your Mind*, Ries and Trout state that "history shows that the first brand in the brain, on the average, gets twice the long-term market share as the Number 2 brand and twice again as much as the Number 3 brand. And the relationships are not easily changed."[3] Both of these concepts — positioning and branding — are fundamental for the development of an effective strategic marketing initiative. Neither is tactical in nature. The development of a strong position and strong branding require time and patience. Repetition of effective communication — often over years — with organizational delivery of promised performance will enable the organization to reach its goals.

Before we can explore the specifics of a strategic marketing plan and its deployment in an IDS, we must understand these two concepts.

WHAT IS POSITIONING AND WHY IS IT IMPORTANT?

Look around you. Everywhere. Noise, noise, noise. We don't mean just loud sounds. We are speaking of the constant bombardment we receive from messages — newspaper ads, Internet ads, television and radio ads, digital and analog billboards, magazines, direct mail, and on and on.

Advertising has to figure out a way to cut through all of that noise and effectively communicate a message about a service or a product. "Positioning is an organized system for finding a window in the mind. It is based on the concept that communication can only take place at the right time and under the right circumstances."[3] This is why research is an important component of strategic marketing. In order to take advantage of the window, we must understand what is in the customer's mind. What is she thinking about our organization? About the competition?

The positioning of the organization contributes to its ability to develop brand loyalty and brand equity. (Both of these concepts are discussed in more detail later in this chapter.) It is important to understand that branding — what distinguishes your organization from others, and what assures your patients (or more broadly, customers) that they have made the right decision — is largely dependent on your positioning in the patients' minds.

Positioning and branding both contribute to the efficacy of word-of-mouth marketing for the organization. In his book, *Patients Build Your Practice*, Michael Cafferky notes that nearly 90 percent of a practice's new patients rely on what others have said about the doctor and that 70 percent of patients rely on family, friends, or other physicians for information about a physician.[4]

HOW DO WE DEVELOP OUR POSITION?

How do we develop the organization's position in the market? Carefully. And thoughtfully. And with knowledge of the market, the customer, and your organization. Because positioning is where your organization rests in the mind of the customer, the process of developing your positioning strategy begins with asking questions and conducting research.

You may decide upon surveys, focus groups, or mystery shoppers. Or a combination of them all. The key is to understand your customers. Understand what they think of your organization and the position it holds for them relative to the competition. (And by the way, take time to find out and understand your competition.)

Once you understand where you stand, you must articulate what position you want to hold and what is unique about what you have to offer. For so long we attempted to differentiate one system from another or one provider from another through claims of quality of care. Our reality today establishes quality as a baseline for all health care. What, then, sets your organization apart? How do you want to be perceived — positioned — in the mind of the customer?

The importance of establishing a clearly articulated positioning objective statement cannot be over-emphasized. The positioning objective becomes the "vision" for the marketing initiative, serving as the backdrop for communication strategies including all forms of advertising, public relations, sponsorship, and special events.

Achieving success in positioning and branding comes with a cost, however. Adequate financial and human resources must be allocated to the process to ensure success. And adequate time must be planned for the efforts to reach fruition

Finally, the organization must deliver on its promise. In the parlance of the day, you must not only talk the talk, but you must, more important, walk the walk. Imagine the IDS seeking to be positioned as one that simplifies the referral process and provides quick and easy access for referring physicians and patients, yet has an automated attendant for its phone system with no less than eight options. The damage done to that organization's position could be irreparable. Failure to provide the promised services at the promised level undermine the brand, reduce brand equity, and all but close the window of opportunity to be positioned in the customer's mind.

WHAT'S YOUR BRAND?

Cleveland Clinic. Mayo Clinic. Oschner Clinic. Each is a brand. Each name creates a picture in the mind of the customer. It's a promise. People are loyal to the brand. They know what to expect. The brand is the symbol for all the organization stands for.

Your brand is you. Or, to be more exact, it is your organization. Remember, your brand wasn't developed overnight. None of the organizations mentioned in this chapter developed their brands overnight. It took years and years of delivering on a promise to create loyal customers willing to spread the good word about the organization.

By developing a strong brand identity you give the customer a simple way to sort through the noise mentioned earlier. You save the customer valuable decision-making time and you assure her of quality through the strength of the brand identity. Your organization is now positioned as brand Number 1 in the mind of the customer — the most enviable place to be.

HOW DO YOU BUILD YOUR BRAND?

Building a brand, or developing brand identity, requires clarity and consistency of your message, delivering on the promise, and repetition in every media form, every customer contact, and every potential customer contact. Brand identity is what your staff looks like, how the phones are answered, the signage, the paperwork, the tone of voicemail prompts, even attention to correct spelling in e-mail messages.

Every action and activity within the scope of an organization's operations contributes to the development of brand identity. Every moment of truth between your organization and your customer and potential customer creates an image in the mind of the customer and contributes to the overall brand identity.

Everything. Everywhere. Everybody. The hospitality industry has learned this well. The better hotels attend to uniforms and scripting of customer-centric situations. The housekeeping staff at these hotels will issue you a "good morning" as you walk down a hallway. Contrast that with a medical practice in which there are no standard uniforms and no standard scripts. And the staff barely acknowledges a patient walking down a hallway.

The brand is a critical part of marketing. Think of focusing on branding and positioning as Hamburger Helper for your marketing initiatives. If the organization has a strong brand identity and strong positioning in the customer's mind, the efficacy of all subsequent marketing efforts is geometrically leveraged.

Our discussion of branding thus far has focused on the external customer. Sartain and Schumann focus on the importance of engaging the employees of the organization in the branding effort and, in fact, in developing an "employer brand."[5]

Let's be clear, it is the staff — the employees of the organization — who interact with the customers at each and every moment of truth. Failure to engage the employees in the brand or a failure of the organization to deliver on its promises to its employees erodes the employees' ability to deliver the brand promise to the customer.[5] Without the employees fully engaged in the "brand," the organization has no chance — no matter how much money is invested — to achieve the positioning or brand identity it seeks.

Branding is for the long term. Branding is not based on episodic transactions, but rather on the development of an identity over time through communications, relationship building, and trust as exhibited by delivering on a promise. We know that behaviorally women put a lot of trust in relationships developed with brands over time. Given the overwhelming role of women in family health care decision making, it only serves to underscore the importance of the development of brand identity for today's market.[6]

WHAT MAKES A SUCCESSFUL MARKETING PROGRAM?

Whether an IDS is large or small, rural or urban, a single location or multiple locations, there are four key factors that contribute to the success of a marketing initiative:

- Focusing on a consumer business orientation;
- Employing a rigorous planning regimen;
- Deploying the program in a controlled manner; and
- Ongoing measurement and monitoring of actual results to planned goals.

We've already discussed the first factor: it is customer-focused. No marketing program can succeed if it is inwardly focused. The customer is the key. The customer is the consumer of health care, and it is the consumer orientation that enables us to keep our focus.

The second component of a successful marketing program is a rigorous and disciplined planning regimen. Marketing is not saying, "I think I'd like to run an ad in the newspaper this week, and oh, let's run an ad on the radio in two weeks." A successful marketing plan has clearly articulated goals and objectives, accountabilities, identification of human resources needs, financial requirements, and a mechanism for evaluation. Planning is a must.

The completed document need not be long, but it should be thoughtful, methodical, and thorough. A truism in organizational strategic planning is that many plans fail in the execution stage. Where the rubber meets the road!

Once the planning has been successfully completed, the deployment of the plan is the third factor, and it is a mission-critical step. A careful, thoughtful deployment is vital to achieve success. The process must be a measured one where timing is of the essence.

The fourth, and final, factor contributing to a successful marketing program is the ongoing measurement and monitoring of actual results to planned goals. Management often states that it cannot manage what it does not measure. In the past, marketing has often been dealt with as a "soft" activity — no specific goals or targets to be achieved, but rather given only a "feel good" or "increase general awareness" goal. Increasing costs in our organizations, increased competition, and declining payments from insurers necessitate a full accounting of the return on investment for the organization's marketing dollars. Marketing tactics should be developed with specific targets and milestones. A measurement process should be in place. And results should be evaluated.

By focusing on a consumer business orientation, employing a rigorous planning regimen, and deploying the program in a controlled manner, the organization dramatically increases its chance for success. With monitoring and measurement along the way, the opportunity for ongoing changes and adjustments in a timely manner is enhanced.

WHAT ARE THE COMPONENTS OF A MARKETING PLAN?

The general format for a marketing plan is similar to that of a business, operations, or strategic plan. The table of contents might look like this:

- Situational analysis and research
- Goals
- Objectives
- Target markets
- Tactics
- Measurement
- Budget
- Evaluation

Let's look at each section separately and explore the content.

Situational analysis and research

This is often called an environmental scan. What is going on in the market? What changes have occurred in the economy, industry, population trends, or demographics? Look outside health care. Understand all of the key factors that have an impact on your market. An excellent source for market information is often a local planning commission.

This is the time to conduct a strengths, weaknesses, opportunities, and threats (SWOT) analysis. Evaluate the internal strengths and weaknesses of the organization, but be sure to focus heavily on the external threats and opportunities.

Consider the use of focus groups. If you haven't conducted one before, there are resources on the Internet and many excellent books available to assist you. If your organization is in a community with a college, inquire to see if there is a business school that can assist you.

Conduct patient surveys, either written or by telephone. Ensure that the survey is well written so as to secure the data in an unbiased fashion.

Mystery shoppers can tell you about your organization. They can highlight access issues, customer service issues, or things being done well.

Time spent in this area of the marketing initiative will pay dividends later in the process. The more factual information available, the less guess work involved in developing the actual marketing plan.

Goals and objectives

What is the organization's goal? What do you hope to achieve? Is it a 7 percent increase in patient volume or the establishment of strong referral patterns for the new occupational medicine program? Be clear. Be specific. Some organizations define goals and objectives separately — others use the terms interchangeably. The important concept is to have clearly articulated targets for performance. It is impossible to evaluate the ultimate success of a program without targets against which to measure.

Ensure that the goals and objectives are SMART. Each should be **s**pecific, **m**easurable, **a**chievable, **r**ealistic, and **t**ime bounded. The key to achievement is having clear and specific goals that can serve as yardsticks to measure performance.

Target markets

The most successful marketing programs take a rifle-shot approach, not a machine-gun approach. No organization has adequate funds to blanket an entire market and sustain the effort for the time necessary to have significant impact.

From your research in the first step of the marketing plan you know what is happening in the market. You have an understanding of your current customer base and have also identified potential new target markets. The goals and objectives established earlier have identified specific milestones in specific areas.

Now is the time to identify the target markets. The more specifically the target markets are defined, the more accurately you can message them. The more narrow the focus, the greater the opportunity for success. The more clearly defined the market, the greater the understanding of the market, the easier it is to develop the appropriate strategy and tactics for deployment.

Tactics

Up to this point the discussion has focused on the strategic components of the marketing plan. The tactical portion of the plan focuses on areas such as packaging, price, promotion, and advertising placement. At this level of the plan, assignments are made on an individual basis with specific measurable goals and timeframes. This is the area in the plan where the success or failure is often determined.

The tactics define the actual implementation and deployment of the strategies into the marketplace. The tactics are the moments of truth we spoke of earlier — the interactions between the organization and the customer during which brand identity and positioning is either enhanced or eroded.

The tactics must be developed consistently with the strategies and mindful of the financial and human resources available within the organization. Underestimating the needs in either category could be detrimental to the ultimate execution of the tactical plan.

Measurement

At this point, strategic goals and objectives have been established. The tactical plan has been developed with specific desired outcomes. Now is the time to develop a plan to measure the success and return on investment of the plan. Numerous techniques are available. Several of them were discussed in the chapter's discussion of the situational assessment and research phase of the marketing plan.

Focus groups provide an excellent source of qualitative information. We can learn about our brand identify from customers. We can determine the positioning of the organization in the mind of the customer. We can bring to the surface underlying issues that may inhibit achievement of our goals.

Patient surveys and telephone calls can identify trends in consumer thinking. Open-ended questions are important to allow for exploration of ideas by the respondent.

If the marketing plan's goals were based on financial or productivity targets, the practice management system and practice accounting system can provide comparative data for measurement. The metrics to be evaluated and the source of data for those metrics must be a part of the plan.

Too many organizations develop a plan and identify metrics to measure achievement and success, but have no idea of where to secure the necessary data for evaluation. Plan in advance. Establish a timetable for the measurement process and adhere to it.

Budget

The budgeting process for the marketing plan benefits from a rigorous discipline. Financial resource requirements must be considered, but so too must human resource requirements. A comprehensive marketing plan often is labor intensive; without adequate staffing the deployment may be undermined.

Marketing budgets vary depending on the organizational structure. Some integrated systems have complete in-house marketing and communications departments, while others may require much of the creative work to be outsourced.

Typical budget categories within a marketing plan might include:

- Brand and logo development;
- Creative and copy writing;

- Production costs for print, direct mail, electronic media;
- Photography or videography;
- Media buy including ad placement and electronic media spots;
- Website development;
- Web hosting and updating;
- Special events and/or sponsorships;
- Special promotions;
- Promotional items; and
- Temporary personnel.

Evaluation

A typical performance improvement cycle includes the development of a plan, the deployment of the plan, the measurement and evaluation, and based on the evaluation either continuation as is, modification, or abandonment.

The evaluation component of the marketing plan and process is critical to both current and future success. The organization must understand the impact of the marketing plan. What was successful? What was not? Why? What have we learned?

Resources are too scarce and the stakes are too high not to fully evaluate the deployment of a strategic marketing initiative. Not only do we want to understand the tangible return on investment, but also it is critical to understand the level of brand identity and positioning of the organization.

This is a time to engage the entire team. A broad spectrum of input can provide invaluable information from distinctly different vantage points. The more that is understood, the better the chances of making improvements for the future.

If strategic goals include the development of a strong brand identity coupled with strong positioning in the market, the marketing efforts must continue over time — often years. As we've already noted this requires ongoing financial and human resources. Understand this well prior to embarking on this initiative.

WHAT ROLE DOES PUBLIC RELATIONS PLAY IN THE MARKETING PLAN?

Public relations is one of the tactics employed in a comprehensive marketing plan. Generally defined as a process to create goodwill about an organization through appropriate messaging, public relations is a low-cost alternative to paid advertising and, due to its nature, carries greater sway with the public.

In the case of paid advertising we can purchase an ad in the print media or a spot in the electronic media and control the message. Contrast that with public relations in which the story is told by a neutral third party — the media — through a news story, interview, or reporting on an event or situation.

Because this exposure is not paid, public relations efforts tend to carry more credibility with the public.

The skill set required for a robust public relations campaign is different than that required for advertising. While both fall under the heading of marketing, each has its own requirements for success.

The public relations area is one in which increased participation from physicians is a prerequisite. The absence of physician participation virtually ensures failure. While we have often found it difficult to secure time from the physicians for interviews during the day, when we have been able to, the results have been impressive.

Being quoted in articles or interviewed on television positions the physician as the expert, the resource for information in the community. No amount of paid advertising can have the same effect.

Public relations is about building relationships over time. Identify and cultivate key media within your community. Don't be seen as the person who always wants something, but rather be known as the person who has valuable information, an interesting story idea, or a hot tip on a new medical issue.

WHAT ARE THE CHALLENGES AND OPPORTUNITIES FOR MARKETING AN INTEGRATED DELIVERY SYSTEM?

Leveraging the brand: vertical integration

Consider this situation: A small community in the Northeast with two hospitals in the community. One hospital is a faith-based organization, and one is a community-owned hospital. The faith-based organization has been in existence for more than 50 years and decides to develop an IDS. The hospital has an excellent reputation in the community — you might say strong brand identity — and is well positioned with patients and non-patients alike.

As practices are integrated into the system, they are allowed to maintain their private practice name, logo, Website, and uniform logos. There is limited to no extension of the hospital brand into the medical practices. The practices elect to keep their appearance of independence, though the fact of employment by the hospital is well known.

We see this as a missed opportunity. The practices fail to receive the benefits from the brand identify of the hospital, and the hospital fails to benefit from the association with the private practices.

Our recommendation for this situation was to leverage the hospital brand for the practices by identifying them as part of the hospital brand, and in turn, benefitting the hospital through the apparent expansion of its access throughout the community. Signage, name tags, paperwork, and lab coats were all modified to tie the practices with the hospital. Benefits were swift and mutual for each of the organizations involved.

This example illustrates the benefits of a marketing plan within a vertically integrated organization. By leveraging the brand — both forward and backward — the IDS and the individual practices each benefit. This is a case in which the benefits of vertical integration can be seen in areas other than clinic operations.

Marketing employed physicians and not independent physician practices

To market employed physicians and not independent physician practices would be the proverbial can of worms, particularly in a small community where options are limited. In the previous section we discussed the benefits to the practice and to the IDS of leveraging the brand and advertising as such. In a small community, that doesn't work so well. In a small community where the non-employed physicians have few options, the potential for anger and animosity between the independent physicians and the IDS is real. Often, physicians object to the IDS advertising its employed physicians and feel that this creates an unfair advantage for those physicians.

The complaint was one of not being able to afford "that" kind of marketing effort, and the potential for loss of patients due to the hospital's advertising alone. In some cases the IDS has provided advertising support through general awareness ads for the independent physicians as well, and in other cases, it has simply indicated to the practices that this was not going to happen. In some instances, other means of providing support to the independent practices were sought by the IDS.

Ultimately the IDS has a fiduciary obligation, among other obligations, to its stakeholders. Prudent business policy suggests that the IDS develop a marketing plan to brand and position the IDS in the marketplace. This is particularly true in a highly competitive marketplace.

CONCLUSION

There is no mystery to developing a successful and comprehensive marketing plan for an IDS. The basic principles of planning and execution apply. A rigorous discipline of consumer-focused thinking will go a long way towards ensuring success.

Careful attention to strategic initiatives and tactical plans ensures thoughtful goals and objectives with a well-developed plan for deployment. We know from experience that the road to ruin is paved with an organization's inability to execute well.

The successful organization and effort will seek to understand its brand identity and positioning in the consumer's mind. Only by thoroughly understanding the mindset of the consumer can the organization develop the necessary strategies and tactics.

This is a process, not a simple transaction. Integrated systems that wish to have successful marketing programs will employ fully the performance improvement system outlined in this chapter: develop the plan, implement or deploy the plan, evaluate, and either adopt it in full, modify it, or abort it. The ability to manage the process is directly tied to the ability to measure performance.

Is there a magic bullet to make a marketing plan work? Yes: accountability at all levels is necessary for success.

REFERENCES

1. E.N. Berkowitz, *Essentials of Health Care Marketing* (Sudbury, MA: Jones and Bartlett Publishers, 2004).
2. Board of Directors, "Definition of Marketing," October 2007. American Marketing Association (January 17, 2009).
3. A. Ries and J. Trout, *Positioning: The Battle for Your Mind* (New York: McGraw-Hill, 1986).
4. M. Cafferky, *Patients Build Your Practice* (New York: McGraw-Hill, 1994).
5. L. Sartain and M. Schumann, *Brand from the Inside* (San Francisco: Jossey-Bass, 2006).
6. M. Gobé, *Emotional Branding: The New Paradigm for Connecting Brands to People* (New York: Allworth Press, 2001).

CHAPTER FOURTEEN

Strategic Planning: What's Next?

Nick A. Fabrizio, PhD, FACMPE, FACHE, and Robert C. Bohlmann, FACMPE

Strategic planning is an important activity in every successful organization, including medical groups. In an integrated delivery system (IDS), it is crucial. Because integrated systems are formed by combining different specialties, different organization types, and different relationships with hospitals and health systems, strategic planning is one of the most important management activities an IDS can perform. It is critical for the newly established or existing IDS to shore up its management team and governance structure to build an effective plan that can address the organization's internal and external strengths, weaknesses, opportunities, and threats (SWOT), and develop both short- and long-term plans. Capturing information in the form of a SWOT analysis, having a structured process to obtain information and communicate that information with internal stakeholders, obtaining consensus on which plans or initiatives to follow, communicating the plan, implementing strategies, and monitoring results are at the heart of effective strategic planning.

Integrated systems that use strategic planning successfully integrate the processes in their management agenda. They perform both formal and informal strategic planning sessions regularly, share the information consistently with leadership and across sites, and most important, commit to revisit and update their strategic plans as a leadership team. Many IDS boards or executive committees devote time at monthly board meetings for updates on strategic goals and initiatives related to those goals. These governing bodies evaluate the progress or limitations toward accomplishing their initiatives so that they can address issues that threaten the successful execution of those plans. It is important for the IDS to have a process to update and refine the organization's current goals, monitor those initiatives, and make course corrections to the implementation plans.

THE INTEGRATION IMPERATIVE: WHY STRATEGIC PLANNING IS SO IMPORTANT

Strategic planning can be thought of as a disciplined effort to produce decisions and actions that guide and shape what the organization is, what it does, and why it does what it does.[1] Many leaders fall into the trap of thinking that a strategic plan must be a static document that covers a multi-year period. They may also have the misconception that the organization must not alter its plans during the time period between formal planning sessions.

Effective strategic planning is a dynamic process that could be altered by changes in both the internal and external environment. Some of these changes could include the loss of providers, the dissolution of an office, the addition of a new group, or the formation of a new relationship with another entity such as a hospital. Other changes may include external forces such as changes in reimbursement, increases in malpractice coverage, changes to compensation plans, and the entry of new competitors in the market or the formation of new relationships with competitors. For these reasons, it is important to have a process with which the board can evaluate the strategic initiatives based on changes in both the internal and external environments. It requires the organization to examine what it is, where it is going, and how it is going to get there.[2]

A strategic plan helps leaders focus on stated and agreed-upon goals within the context of the internal and external environment. Strategic planning also helps the organization to focus on its most crucial issues and challenges. Given this framework, leaders must decide on the direction the IDS is heading and the resources needed to compete and thrive as an integrated system.

Is your organization confused as to where it is going? Does your board know where it wants to go? Do physicians and managers have disagreements as to the direction the organization is heading? Are you surprised about how you got into your current situation? Do you often wonder whether fate or luck is steering your practice? If the answer to any of these questions is yes, use the organizational pre-planning self-assessment shown in Exhibit 14.1 to determine how strategic planning can work for you.

STRENGTHS AND WEAKNESSES IN THE PLANNING APPROACH

Integrated systems can improve the planning process by taking advantage of the strengths and weaknesses of each party in the organization: hospital leaders, medical practice leaders, physicians, and other managers and staff. Typically, hospital and IDS leaders are trained in business school to take a team approach to decision making. Working with and through people to accomplish objectives is taught, respected, and developed. Hospital and IDS leaders are taught that working with and through people is their most important leadership skill — it is what separates good from great leaders. As such, hospitals typically are good at strategic planning. They tend to create well-thought-out and well-researched short- and long-term goals that match their human and financial resources in accomplishing objectives.

Many large hospitals and health systems have their own strategic planning departments or leaders who spend all or most of their time linking short- and long-term objectives to business, operating, and marketing plans. These institutions also use both simple and elaborate tracking tools to implement, monitor, and report on plan objectives. They have worked their plans into

EXHIBIT 14.1 ■ Strategic Planning Readiness Assessment

Check the box that best captures your group's readiness to create a meaningful strategic plan.

1. Do you have a directed strategy with delineated goals? ☐ Yes ☐ No
2. Do you monitor your strategy regularly and list your progress, shortcomings, and develop action plans to address those areas in need? ☐ Yes ☐ No
3. Do you have an effective governance structure? ☐ Yes ☐ No
4. Has your group ever scheduled a formal planning meeting? ☐ Yes ☐ No
5. Do you have a mission, vision, and values statement? ☐ Yes ☐ No
6. Do you have external issues or forces that require major attention? ☐ Yes ☐ No
7. Do you have internal issues that you never talk about or act upon? ☐ Yes ☐ No
8. Have your physicians ever dedicated one-on-one time to discuss their plans? ☐ Yes ☐ No
9. Have you ever used a trained facilitator experienced in health care who was focused on delivering a strategic plan linked to strategic initiatives? ☐ Yes ☐ No
10. Do you have an existing strategic plan that lists your goals and actions, and identifies a responsible person charged with carrying out those objectives? ☐ Yes ☐ No
11. Have you carefully mapped out your short-term and long-term plans matching your desires with your institutional commitments? ☐ Yes ☐ No
12. Have you dedicated resources to your strategic initiatives? ☐ Yes ☐ No
13. Have you identified your strengths, weaknesses, opportunities, and threats? ☐ Yes ☐ No
14. Is the competition impacting your practice? ☐ Yes ☐ No
15. Do you make your strategic initiatives part of your operating and business plans? ☐ Yes ☐ No
16. Do your staff and all of your key stakeholders understand your strategic initiatives? ☐ Yes ☐ No

Count the YES Responses. TOTAL NUMBER OF YES RESPONSES = ____________

Scoring Key:

13–16 "YES": You have a strategically oriented group and have already dedicated the time, resources, and commitment necessary to move your strategic plans to strategic initiatives. You may only need to refine your existing plans to take advantage of the competitive landscape and position your group to be the leader in an existing or new service line. You may also need to address your succession plans to ensure that you stay on top.

9–12 "YES": You have a baseline commitment to strategic planning and need some fine-tuning to bring your group from strategic plans to realizing the benefits of effective strategic initiatives.

5–8 "YES": It's time to revisit your group's goals and reason for existence. You will need to ready your group for creating a management framework designed to focus on long-term strategies instead of decision making on the fly. It's time to prepare by capitalizing on your strengths and correcting your weaknesses. You will need to determine how leadership will advance and support the strategic planning agenda.

0–4 "YES": What are you waiting for? It is time to begin formulating a timetable to discuss the importance of strategic planning with your leadership group and physicians. You must develop a plan, which will ensure your long-term survival. Group buy-in and a commitment to business planning are the hallmarks for your success.

the leadership agenda and have regular meetings with hospital leadership to discuss plans and any limitations or opportunities created as a result of the planning process.

In contrast, physicians are trained to be independent thinkers and use data quickly to assess, manage, and treat patients. When we are sick, we rely on our physician to give us immediate answers to our questions without consulting a team. At times, our physicians need to refer us to certain specialists, but even with up to two or three separate consultations, they will diagnose over 98 percent of our ailments in a relatively short period of time. As patients, we would not appreciate our physician telling us that she needs to consult with a team that meets monthly over the course of a year or so before giving us the answers to our medical problems. In the business world, this skill set of the physicians is useful for independent and quick decision making — situations where one does not rely on a team approach. Thus, physicians by training and temperament tend to have decision-making skills tailored to short-term planning needs.

The most successful integrated systems use the strengths of each stakeholder: physicians and other medical practice leaders for decisions that require quick, decisive action based on data, and hospital leaders when decisions require careful planning and consensus. Recognizing the importance of gathering information quickly and making concrete but immediate plans that show signs of improvements is as important as creating careful and deliberate plans that bring others into the process to be involved, invested, and part of longer-term plans and successes.

One of the most successful strategies that several integrated systems use is to place physicians on project teams where short-term decisions and implementation plans are needed. These assignments also help build credibility into the process so that physicians may see that their opinions and suggestions are leading to positive change or actions for the IDS. However, it is important that if physicians serve on the management team or board, they learn the importance, and often be trained in, the team approach to management. Care must be taken to help physicians serving on the management team or board to learn the value of longer term planning and the processes involved in creating, fostering, and building support for long-term plans or projects.

CAPACITY AND COMPETITION

Because health care and the delivery of health care are not static, an IDS must continually assess its capacity for delivering services. The IDS must determine the extent to which it has the ability, through its providers, ancillaries, and health facilities, to deliver the needed services in relation to the demand and price for those services. Several factors affect this relationship:

- The ability to recruit and retain the necessary professionals;
- The ability to purchase and provide needed ancillary services; and
- The quality and attractiveness of its physical facilities.

▪ CASE STUDY ▪

What Is the Value of Status?

Ladera Health System invested in obtaining a high profile, but may end up in last place anyway

Ladera Health System (LHS) is a 500-bed hospital located in a Midwestern city with a population of approximately 750,000 and a potential health care market of twice that size. Until the early 2000s, LHS had deferred consideration of making the transition into the IDS domain.

In 2005, LHS was approached by several subspecialty group practices interested in affiliation. LHS was an attractive affiliation partner because it was recognized as the premier quality and service-oriented institution of the three hospitals in the city. Two specialty groups affiliated with LHS the following year and a third in 2007. The affiliations gave LHS strong integrated services in cancer care, cardiology, and gastroenterology, and a total of 17 physicians.

LHS administration was not savvy in dealing with practice management issues and employed physician staff relations. The system further found that the practice affiliations were capital intensive. The cash position of the newly acquired practices was compromised by less-than-effective revenue cycle management.

Simultaneous with LHS's integration activity, both of its competitors — the two other hospitals in town — launched initiatives to acquire medical practices, but concentrated their efforts on primary care.

LHS, because of its reputation, became attractive to a number of smaller primary care groups, both within the city proper but also on the city's rural periphery. Several of these groups approached LHS to propose their acquisition.

Instead of being receptive to primary care affiliation, LHS administration took the position that they had their hands full managing the three specialty practices already acquired and, further, LHS lacked the capital to assimilate more money-losing practices. LHS administration also tended to be less than diplomatic in turning away other prospective acquisition candidates.

As might be anticipated, most of the turned-down practices, which were already "psyched up" about the affiliation concept, were wooed by the other two hospital-based systems in town.

By 2008 it became apparent that admissions to LHS's specialists were declining because of altered primary care physician loyalties. Having missed the opportunity to assimilate well-established practices, LHS was required to recruit and initiate its own primary care practice locations — a very slow and expensive proposition.

By mid-2008, LHS's market-dominant position for its flagship services was showing a decline in income and volume of services. This erosion could have been easily avoided by a more progressive practice orientation. Within a three-year period, LHS's market position was a shadow of its former self. Conversely, competing subspecialty practices, although remaining independent but now loyal to the other hospitals, benefited and prospered, as did as the institutions themselves.

For example, if an IDS has a hospital with an old infrastructure, outdated ancillary equipment, and inefficient workflow processes, it will not be as appealing to the community or to other physicians who use those services.

The presence in the community of more appealing facilities from competitors could weaken the market position for the IDS. For example, if the integrated system's labor and delivery floor was built in the 1960s, it is probably not set up to be efficient in today's environment — the expectations of providers and mothers-to-be were not the same then as they are now. In addition to seeking a more efficient design, obstetricians and other providers involved in deliveries use hospital "birthing centers" much differently today than they did in the 1960s. As a result, it is hard for these older and often unrenovated hospitals to compete with newer facilities in terms of efficiency.

Newer facilities also offer superior marketing and customer service advantages. An effective strategic planning process will allow the IDS to know what steps it must take to keep up with changes in technology and facility design. This planning will not only improve the IDS's competitive advantage but also will increase its ability to market services, keep patients using the services provided within the IDS, and capture market share.

KEY PRE-REQUISITES AND PREVIOUS PLANS

While having no strategic plan, or one that is outdated, is a recipe for underperformance, having many plans that fail to mesh also is a hazard. One of the first steps an IDS must take in developing its strategic vision is to gather together all of the separate strategic, business, operating, and marketing plans of its various units. As an IDS grows and adds more units, each will likely bring along its own "strategies for success." Because there may be many separate practices and hospitals combined into an IDS, the board of the IDS must review those plans to see how, or if, each individual plan fits into the entire plan. This is an easier task if the IDS has a strategic plan to start with.

If the organization does not have a strategic plan, its board must inform the leaders of the medical groups and other entities that have strategic plans that they will be important members in the development of an organization-wide strategic plan. They also should be told that any individual plans or strategic initiatives will need IDS board approval prior to the commitment of funds and personnel. These leaders should be assured that this does not mean that strategic plans of the IDS–owned groups will be eliminated, but it does mean that the IDS organization will need to be involved in directing such plans. All of the entities within the IDS must be aware that the IDS will have one strategic plan and that each office, facility, and unit will play an important part within that plan; they will be expected to develop strategic initiatives or plans that are related to the organizational plan.

If the organization has several different departments or specialties under its umbrella, can they each have their own strategic plan? This is a difficult question to address. Rather than getting caught up in the definition of "strategic plan," the IDS should set a clear path: there is one master strategic plan for the IDS. If groups within the IDS desire to have their own strategic plans or initiatives, they must relate those plans and initiatives to — and not be at odds with — the master plan.

Often, individual departments within a hospital or large single specialty or multi-specialty groups within an IDS have strategic initiatives or plans that they should roll into the master IDS plan. This task is relatively easy if one links the separate plans or initiatives in a Microsoft Excel file and then links that file with the master IDS file. Think of these plans as separate rows on an Excel spreadsheet. The organization would have the same or standard columns that track the project or initiative, person responsible, start and end dates, and so on, and then different rows of information that can include the initiatives from the other specialties, locations, or departments.

THE BOARD'S RESPONSIBILITY IN PLANNING

In regard to strategic planning, the IDS board is responsible for establishing, measuring, monitoring, and allocating funds. It also is responsible for holding people accountable for accomplishing the objectives delineated in the strategic plan.

An effective board should be comprised of a mix of both administrative and physician leaders who are representative of the entire organization. These leaders should have their pulse on the organization and be able to understand the needs of the individual clinics and departments of the IDS in decision making. This does not mean that every clinical department must be represented. However, one of the most important tasks for these leaders, especially physician leaders on the board, is to establish effective communication channels with the breadth of physicians and specialties represented by the IDS. As such, both physician and non-physician leaders should hold meetings that solicit input from all of the different specialties within the IDS. While this may seem like a time-consuming task, it is! It is also one of the most important tasks in building credibility and getting the pulse of the departments that make up the organization. This information-gathering will pay dividends when it's time for strategic planning.

The board must also determine which of its members will meet with certain departments and how often. A meeting schedule must be established so that the individual clinics or departments have a chance to work with board members to discuss their concerns and ideas for improving the organization. This dialogue is also important so that each physician and each clinic and department sees that the IDS's leaders care about and seek their involvement in the IDS, and understand the issues at both the 30,000-foot level and at ground zero.

Once this dialogue between the board and individual groups is established, which often comes in the form of quarterly meetings with the individual clinics, administrative (non-physician) personnel can be dedicated to working with the groups to establish their individual strategic initiatives. Some individual clinics may be large enough to have the personnel to support their own professional managers who could be charged with gathering information, facilitating meetings, and working with the IDS to establish and coordinate these strategic planning initiatives into the master strategic plan.

Once these individual or departmental plans are rolled up into a comprehensive strategic plan, the board is responsible for measuring and monitoring this master plan against stated and documented objectives. The board must continually measure outcomes related to the plans and make course corrections along the way. Monitoring the strategic plan should be a regular part of the board agenda.

At least every month, the board should review one objective or goal from the strategic plan and ensure that the medical group or department is on track toward accomplishing that objective. Exhibit 14.2 illustrates a sample executive summary grid that the board can use to help facilitate these review meetings. This executive summary grid should list each goal, the status of that goal, the person responsible for the goal(s), timelines, and the percentage completed. The board members should be prompted to ask tough questions during these review sessions. After working so hard to develop the goals, board members should be expected to take a close and critical view of where the goals are in relation to the resources used and the amount of progress (preferably expressed as a percentage of the goal that has been completed). If the status of an objective is unclear, the board should ask for further information. If the status of that objective is poor, the board may invite the person responsible for that objective to present that initiative along with the progress or lack thereof related to that objective at the next board meeting.

By spending a little time at every meeting on one goal or strategic initiative, the board can more easily accomplish addressing the plan in its entirety and resolve necessary issues in a timely fashion. The board should spend time quarterly taking a more formal role in reviewing the strategic plan by dedicating a significant portion of that meeting on the overall IDS strategic plan.

EXHIBIT 14.2 ■ Executive Action Item Grid

Goal Number	Start Date	Person Accountable	Deadline	% Complete	Comments/ Resources

LEADERSHIP FOCUS

In a study by Eric Beinhocker and Sarah Kaplan, one of the major limitations observed in building effective strategic plans was a failure by top leaders to dedicate enough time to the strategic planning process.[3] According to their study of 30 companies, including Boeing, Coca-Cola, GE, IBM, Intel, Johnson & Johnson, Microsoft, and Motorola, the majority of the chief executive officers interviewed wanted to spend about a third of their time on strategy. These executives wanted to focus their efforts on organizational, divisional, and departmental goals.

Related to the health care field, one can easily imagine that in a large organization such as an IDS, strategic thinking could easily consume half of the leadership's time. It is important to then think of strategic planning as strategic thinking in order to relay the importance of strategic planning as a disciplined management task. It is up to every organization to develop its own management tools or scorecards that can be used to keep the organization on track in developing and monitoring those initiatives.

PHYSICIAN INVOLVEMENT IN PLANNING

The IDS medial director plays a crucial role in strategic planning. This leader must endorse the process and continue to be involved in various steps of the strategic planning process. The medical director must continually discuss the merits of the strategic planning process with other physicians within the IDS. The medical director must not only have an open door policy with IDS physicians, he or she must also routinely meet with the various medical practice leaders to discuss their individual group's performance, operations, and strategic goals as they relate to the IDS's strategic plan. By meeting with the individual groups, the IDS medical director is also in a better position to uncover trends and early indicators to looming problems. More importantly, by meeting with other physician leaders, the IDS medical director has the ability to mentor and identify future physician leaders.

All of the physician members of an IDS should be involved with strategic planning. The organization should gather its senior leaders periodically, at least once per year, for a strategic planning retreat during which the leaders can discuss where the organization is in relation to its stated goals and discuss course correction strategies. The physicians should be active members in the planning process and should be responsible for strategic activities in the planning process.

In addition, the medical director, along with the medical director for each specialty practice, should be responsible for creating an environment in which the physicians and providers within that group are solicited for input. Input comes from both face-to-face discussions when there is a manageable number of interviewees and through written surveys when face-to-face discussions are not feasible. The IDS should create standard questions based on gathering information related to the strengths, weaknesses, opportunities, and threats (SWOT) of the individual departments and groups. Physicians should be asked where they see their group in 1 year and in 3 years, along with targeted questions depending on the local issues affecting health care in that community. This survey information should be sent to a central location, tabulated, and shared with the IDS board of directors. This information should also be quantified to better support and create both IDS and individual strategic plans.

FACING THE FUTURE

Effective strategic planning can better help to prepare integrated systems of all types and structures to change, adapt, and lead their respective health care systems through the next decade. The relationships that medical groups have with each other, hospitals, health systems, academic departments, health departments, and state governments will continue to evolve over the coming years. Developing effective relationships with these constituents requires an IDS to understand and actively manage the strategic planning process within its institution. Integrated systems must have dedicated resources for strategic planning and make this process part of their culture. The resources needed to effectively plan for the future include political awareness, expertise, financial resources, personnel, commitment from the leadership team, and the ability to execute those plans.

WHAT'S NEXT: THE HOT BUTTONS

There is a tendency for any organization, upon accomplishment of a major strategic initiative, to step back and assume the position, "We did it — we're now all set for the future — let's sit back and be proud!" Sadly, this attitude typically occurs after a health system has completed its first round of medical practice integration. This complacency may last for a few months, or even a couple of years, until bumps in the integration road begin to appear, such as dissention, loss of a group, or other problems. These events usually result in a wake-up call in which leaders say, "We should have thought of that!" and echoed by IDS physicians asking, "Why didn't those people in the leadership suite see that coming?"

Like a good general looking at the next battle when mopping up the current engagement, IDS management should proactively anticipate and avoid future land mines or, more importantly, recognize opportunities before the competition does. It is incumbent upon IDS leaders and their board of directors to both anticipate the obstacles and opportunities of the immediate future, and strategize in advance to project ultimate potential achievement over the longer term.

The hot buttons, or most apparent needs of an IDS, appear to be generalized within the following categories:

- How big should we be? What size is optimum?
- What are our recruiting priorities?
- What are the dangers of refusing affiliation to an interested physician practice?
- Do we have sufficient resource data to make intelligent decisions?

▪ CASE STUDY ▪

How Big Should We Be?

This IDS knew the right questions to ask, but didn't have enough data to get the right answers.

Alpine View Memorial Hospital (AVMH) is an IDS located in a growing mid-sized city in the Southwest. It consists of a flagship facility and three community hospitals operating in regional towns. AVMH "had done it right" in the opinion of its administration, board of directors, and outside consultant. It successfully integrated and recruited a staff of more than 150 physicians, consisting of 110 primary care and 40 medical and surgical specialists. The primary care practices were positioned throughout AVMH's service area, creating a patient admission conduit within a very competitive market. AVMH's competition consisted of an equal-sized system within its primary city and another larger system located in an adjacent city that attracted market share from the northern and western periphery of AVMH's main service area.

AVMH's IDS had achieved a reasonably mature stature over several decades. Its administration, supported by the board, had developed a proactive, participatory relationship with its physician staff. The physicians generally felt well-respected working within a market-competitive compensation system. Financial performance, in terms of funded loss, was well within the median for similar systems reported in the Medical Group Management Association's (MGMA) annual Cost Survey. AVMH, with its physician coverage and quality service orientation, had been able to negotiate favorable payer contracts for both its inpatient and outpatient services.

With everything seemingly in place and respectful system financial margins, many integrated systems would tend to relax, but that attitude did not reconcile with AVMH's leadership. Looking ahead, leadership raised questions in anticipation of strategic planning:

- How big should our physician staff be? How many physicians and what specialties do we need?
- Can we depend upon non-employed specialists for continued support?
- If non-employed physicians ask to affiliate with us but we turn them down, what will happen to our relationship with them?

AVMH's planning orientation boiled down to two basic but multi-faceted issues. The first issue was to quantify a balance between existing hospital capacity and the patient volume needed to fill that capacity and origin of that volume. The second issue, but one of equal importance, was to identify the service line necessary to maintain the system's competitive position in the market. Service line dependency, as it relates to physician staff, in turn, recognized specialty depth and optimum size necessary for coverage and practice efficiency. Service capacity is also of particular concern to prevent patient out-migration seeking access or perceived better quality.

In attempting to address both issues — how to balance current capacity with volume and how to identify services needed to compete — the system's strategic planning efforts hit a

(Case Study continues on next page)

snag when leaders realized that there was limited admitting information to review. Good census data attributed to admitting physicians were readily available, but secondary-level data identifying the primary sources of patients were not. Data regarding patient referrals by AVMH–employed primary care physicians to specialists, who then admitted those patients to the hospital, were not available. There was no way within the existing system to track patients from primary care physicians to specialists (in some cases, to several specialists) and then to either inpatient or outpatient departments of the system's hospitals. In the absence of data, AVMH planning was restricted to rather limited estimates.

The matter became further complicated when addressing service line capacity because many specialties referring the AVMH facilities also had loyalties to non–AVMH hospitals. Most of these were private practice, single-specialty groups.

AVMH's primary challenge was clearly the development of an internal tracking system on which it could accurately determine the influence of its employed physician base.

This example emphasizes that strategic planning is not entirely oriented to external market-related objectives, but must also recognize the limitations of internal capacity to support the plan's objectives. As the hospital/medical practice integration movement accelerates, a corollary trend will be an emphasis on territorial turf and establishing primary care catchment areas. Service areas will be less defined in metro areas as practice sites will tend to have overlapping catchment areas. On the other hand, clear lines of market definition will exist between metro areas. Although medical practices in peripheral areas may not have strong loyalties to any one system or hospital, those loyalties could be enhanced through outreach efforts.

AVMH established its planning work within an ill-defined time line, because it recognized that its competition was, in all probability, also in a planning mode.

- Are capital resources adequate to achieve optimum size?
- Who leads the IDS? What should be the physician's role?
- What is our culture? Are all the pieces within the IDS bonding and going in the same direction?
- Do we need a new brand to designate an integrated entity?

Strategic planning efforts, to be realistic, must not only consider external opportunities and anticipate environmental changes, but also evaluate the internal capacity necessary to achieve the desired goals. As history has demonstrated, many battles initiated by visionary leaders have been lost because of internal logistical limitations or by not being sufficiently nimble to adjust tactics in the face of adversity or unforeseen opportunities.

It is not unusual for management of growth organizations, particularly those adjusting to new business lines, to remain focused on that which is comfortable and, therefore, pay less attention to or ignore their most recent acquisitions. This thesis has been repeatedly demonstrated by health care systems.

As discussed earlier in this chapter, it is also not unusual to observe hospitals with a major integration strategy to completely ignore physician leaders from their acquired groups when it comes to strategic planning. This not only is unfortunate but also is actually a reversal of direction when the strategy was initially predicated upon IDS development and gaining the advantages of the physician practices who initiate medical care and orchestrate patient service throughout the IDS.

REFERENCES

1. J. M. Bryson, *Strategic Planning for Public and Nonprofit Organizations: A Guide to Strengthening and Sustaining Organization Achievement* (San Francisco: Jossey-Bass, 1995).

2. N. Fabrizio, *Goals into Gold: Strategic Planning for Health Care Professionals* (Englewood, CO: Medical Group Management Association, 2008).

3. E. Beinhocker and S. Kaplan, "Tired of Strategic Planning?" *The McKinsey Quarterly, Special Edition on Strategy* (2002): 48–57.

APPENDIX

IDS Affiliation Feasibility Discussion Checklist

The first step in determining whether or not a medical practice should consider strategic and financial alignment with a hospital should be to conduct a feasibility study. During this step the medical practice should set forth and amplify strategic objectives to support the practice's integration with the hospital. The practice should also inquire "are there any arrangements falling short of a full integration?"

When initiating integration discussions, it is important for a medical group to identify all questions necessary to support a decision. Most affiliation problems are typically attributed to misunderstandings related to expectations and later introduction of major considerations, which should have been identified in the first place.

The discussion points are listed as follows:

1. **Organizational structure.** In response to the practice being integrated as a division within the hospital system, how will the organization relate and function?
   - Spell out the practice's responsibility, authority, and reporting.
   - Identity the hospital's control points ("reserve powers").
2. **Practice valuation.** What will be included and what will be the purchase arrangements?
   - What and how will assets be valued?
   - How will debt be assumed?
   - With respect to real estate, will this be a purchase or lease, what will be the terms, and how will the values or rate be established?
3. **Board of directors.** Will any practice physician or executive have a seat on the hospital or system board?

4. **Physician employment.** Specific factors include:
   - Compensation system — spell this out.
   - Compensation cap — several physicians are very high producers with justified high compensation. Will there be any limitation?
   - Will recruiting and physician practice compensation guarantees be assumed by the hospital?
   - Benefit structure — spell this out.
   - Vesting and longevity — will there be a credit for the practice's employment time (longevity)?
   - Protection against future change or compensation reduction. A down-side protection relationship should be established. Medical Group Management Association (MGMA) survey data would represent an industry indicator.
5. **Clinical support staff.** Will existing positions related to supporting physicians remain?
6. **Hours, days, coverage.** Will there be any change to current physician scheduling?
7. **Practice loss (red ink).** It is important to clarify "loss" items from the beginning:
   - Identify hospital line items, which may be included in the general and administrative overhead assigned to the practice division.
   - Identify the current contribution (direct profit and overhead gains) of ancillary departments.
8. **Termination options.** Specific factors include:
   - No area prohibitions for physicians returning to private practice.
   - Spell out specific conditions for separation (such as financial, malpractice insurance, etc.).
9. **Geographic practice restrictions.** Will specialists and primary care be restricted within particular service areas? (This includes pediatrics, pulmonology, nephrology, and other specialties to be identified. These specialties currently serve outreach areas, and any limitation will be financially adverse to the physicians, as well as the hospital.)
10. **Practice nonphysician staff.** Specific factors include:
    - Identify any positions that will not be absorbed.
    - Confirm wage and salary levels (will there be a change?).
    - Identify benefits.
    - Will the practice's longevity carry forward with respect to benefit applications?
    - It is assumed that ancillary departments will be consolidated. Can the practice's technicians be assimilated by the hospital?

11. **Consolidation of existing hospital physician/provider staff (those already employed) under the physician division (practice) structure.** How will this be done?

12. **Practice management system.** Will the existing system be retained or discontinued? Is revenue cycle management to be separate or consolidated within the hospital? Recommend separation.

13. **EMR.** Will the existing system be retained or discontinued? Recommend separation. Will paper records be retained within the offices or centralized?

14. **Physician termination policy.** Identify specific details related to termination or penalties that exist now or may be added in the future.

15. **Non-executive/HR policy.** Define the terms.

16. **Meeting requirements.** Identify meeting requirements for physician and nonphysician staff. (Some IDS requirements are excessive.)

17. **Malpractice coverage.** Identify carrier and limits and other applicable requirements.

18. **Quality and service measurements.** Do, or will, quality and service measurements apply in any respect?

19. **Ancillary service access points.** Identify ancillary service access points (patient and provider convenience).

20. **Dispute resolution procedures.** Establish procedures for resolving disputes.

21. **Go/no-go limit.** In the event that a segment of the practice's physician staff would elect not to integrate. Is there a go/no-go limit within "doing a deal?"

22. **Outside income.** Is there an outside income policy?

23. **Physician ownership/participation arrangements.** If there are physician ownership/participation arrangements in medical-related joint ventures, etc., will there be an immediate or future issue?

24. **Transition time.** If consolidation takes place, the practice will have a six-month, rather intense wind-down responsibility, typically followed by declining responsibility. Can an arrangement be made to allow assimilated staff employees to accomplish this transition activity?

About the Author/Editor

Nick A. Fabrizio, PhD, FACMPE, FACHE, is a principal consultant with the Medical Group Management Association (MGMA) Health Care Consulting Group and a member of the faculty at Cornell University in the Sloan Program in Health Administration. Nick has been an administrator of a medical practice and managed ambulatory practices for a community hospital. He is the author of the MGMA-published book *Goals into Gold: Strategic Planning for Health Care Professionals* (2007) and the co-developer of the Integrated Delivery Roundtable™, www.idsrountable.com.

Nick has more than 15 years of practice management and health system experience in private physician and large medical group practices, for-profit and non-profit hospitals and health systems, academic medical centers, physician faculty practice plans, as well as ambulatory care networks. His primary expertise is in physician practice management and managing complex physician–hospital relationships and clinical enterprises in a broad range of environments. This experience includes helping align the interests of physicians and hospitals to optimize business and operational performance while achieving financial, quality, service, and market goals.

Nick has served a variety of clients throughout the United States, including medical groups ranging from 1 to more than 800 physicians, community hospitals, and national hospital systems. He has also worked with several integrated delivery systems, faith-based systems, for-profit and not-for-profit foundation medical practices, and management service organizations.

About the Contributors

Robert C. Bohlmann, FACMPE, has been a principal consultant with the MGMA Health Care Consulting Group since 1984 and was the group's first director. In his more than 30 years of experience in medical group practice administration, he has served more than 500 medical groups, hospitals, and integrated systems in 48 states, helping them with strategic planning, physician compensation, conflict resolution, and operational and financial performance.

Cynthia L. Dunn, RN, FACMPE, is a senior consultant with the MGMA Health Care Consulting Group. Cindy has more than 30 years of experience in health care, including administrator of private medical practices nursing management for a hospital-owned physician practice. She has managed technology implementation, medical office and ambulatory surgery center planning and construction, as well as frequently facilities strategic planning meetings.

Richard D. Hansen, MS, is vice president and managing principal of the MGMA Health Care Consulting Group. His more than 30 years of experience in health care management include practice administrator for single and multispecialty group practices and vice president of two California hospitals. As a consultant, he has worked with more than 300 medical groups, helping them facilitate change, establish strategic direction, and develop and recruit executive leadership.

Kenneth T. Hertz, CMPE, a principal with the MGMA Health Care Consulting Group, has 30 years of management experience in leadership positions at small and large health care organizations, including primary care, multispecialty, and large integrated systems. Ken has won numerous advertising and marketing awards during his career and was the recipient of the 2005 Edward B. Stevens Article of the Year Award awarded by MGMA.

W. David Holloway, MD, CPE, FAAFP, is senior vice president and chief medical officer for Salem Health, a growing two-hospital system in Salem, Oregon. Areas of responsibility include Salem Health's innovative Center for Patient Safety and Clinical Effectiveness, Surgical Services, Medical Staff

Services, and the employed Physician Practices. Past experience includes development of integrated physician groups within multi-hospital systems as well as serving four years as Chief Quality Officer for Parkview Health. Special interests include developing physician leaders and systematically improving the reliability of processes in complex environments.

Lisa Holloway, MA, put her master's degree in organizational communication to work for many years as a continuing education director for Tulsa (Oklahoma) Community College. She now enjoys doing volunteer work and helping her husband with professional projects as needed.

Bruce A. Johnson, JD, MPA, is a consultant and health care attorney with experience in health care business and regulatory compliance for physician organizations. He also is a partner in the health law practice group of Faegre & Benson, LLP, in Denver. Bruce has extensive experience in the application of Medicare and Medicaid fraud and abuse, Stark self-referral prohibitions, antitrust law, and other legal issues. He is coauthor of the MGMA-published book *Physician Compensation Plans* (2006) and co-developer of the Integrated Delivery Roundtable™, www.idsrountable.com.

Trip Kinmon, FACMPE, is a consultant with the MGMA Health Consulting Group. His more than 37 years of experience include senior management positions in virtually every sector of the health care industry — from multispecialty and single-specialty group practices to integrated delivery and academic-affiliated practices. Trip has extensive experience in assisting groups develop and implement strategic plans and identify areas of growth opportunities. He has a special interest in physician–hospital relationships, especially in rural settings.

Rosemarie Nelson, MS, a principal with the MGMA Health Care Consulting Group, consults with health care organizations and conducts educational seminars on health care technology and operations. She is nationally recognized for her contributions and expertise in the field of information technology. Rosemarie has been a medical office manager and she has managed project implementation teams as well as software engineers in the design, implementation, and training of medical practice software.

Index

In this index "*ex*" refers to exhibits.

T

U

V

W